MY ADVENTURE WITH LUPUS—

Living with a Chronic Illness

Robert L. Yocum

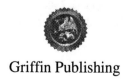

Griffin Publishing

First Edition 1995
10 9 8 7 6 5 4 3 2 1

ISBN   1-882180-45-3

Griffin Publishing books are available at quantity discounts with bulk purchase for education, business, or sales promotional use. Contact Publishing Specials Sales by writing or fax.

Published by
Griffin Publishing
544 West Colorado Street
Glendale California 91204
(818) 244-2128 (818) 242-1172 Fax
Manufactured in the United States of America

Contents

Foreword

Last week a stressed-out man sat in my office describing his chronic headaches, which began after an injury. His medicine wasn't helping, and worse, his doctor could find no organic cause, so he recommended psychotherapy. I was also consulted by a woman who has been treated for cancer and other major organic illnesses. Her stress level from fear of a new outbreak of some major illness at every ache and pain had driven her into depression and hopelessness. She was also told to consult with a mental health therapist to help decrease her anxiety. They wanted something practical and within their reach. I had just read the manuscript of My Adventure With Lupus by Robert Yocum and found myself better prepared to empathize and offer strategies for empowerment, and a sense of meaning to these individuals. I believe it will become an excellent resource to others as well.

Bob Yocum, a victim of chronic lupus, advocates the possibility of turning tragedy into adventure. This goes beyond merely enduring one's suffering with a good attitude. Bob chooses to see in his condition a unique opportunity for growth and further expansion of life, rather than focusing on its limitation and pain. He discusses the importance of support groups, of including family and friends in the educational process, and of self-powerment. He stresses the growth of new skills in communication and collaborative decision-making with your doctor and other professionals on your treatment team.

Bob also believes in the development of a healthy personality through self management strategies, such as humor, the healthy grieving process, self-discipline, and the avoidance of adrenaline addiction. Throughout his book, Bob's faith in Jesus Christ, and faith-centered lifestyle is considered foundational as he addresses some of the most troublesome questions shared by patients with chronic illness, such as: "why am I not miraculously healed?" and, "why me?"

Like so many other lupus patients, Bob has been a high achiever all of his life. As an energetic youth he enjoyed the rigors of ranch life. As a wild young man he raced motorcycles, then fought for his country in the South Pacific during World War II, surviving torpedoes and kamikazes. Later, having undergone a spiritual transformation, he found a good wife and invested his energies and talents in Christian ministry, building new churches.

About thirty years ago, when I met Bob, he pastored the local Baptist church a few blocks from my home. I was a high-school student at that time, interested in both theology and psychology (but more often his daughter, Audrey). Bob always had time for me, and he always had something worthwhile to add to my life. He would open my mind to a certain topic, often engaging me in friendly debate, then loaning me an appropriate book. In subsequent discussions Bob would make sure that I had read the book and acquired its essential wisdom.

I recall Bob's entry into the wilderness of chronic, debilitating illness. Pastoring a shrinking white congregation in an area undergoing rapid racial change, Bob also worked full-time as a motorcycle mechanic. When his narrow-thinking denomination told him he was too old to take another pastorate, Bob entered the secular marketplace and rose quickly to the top as an industrial tool salesman. Amidst this success, the "wolf" (lupus) began attacking, forcing early retirement.

Today Bob continues his struggle, having outlived the medical-odds doomsayers, having grown wiser from his battles with the disease. He remains an active learner, a talented teacher and an unselfish friend to others in need. He has written this book from a practical viewpoint acquired through experience. It is a warm and interesting book with something worthwhile to say. I recommend it to my fellow helping professionals and to all who experience some form of chronic suffering.

Michael R. League,
Licensed Marriage, Family and Child Counselor

Acknowledgments

The help and encouragement others have given me while writing this book is deeply appreciated. Especially the encouragement and support that Jana Deem, a lupus patient, has given from time to time when I have asked for her opinions on what I have written is appreciated.

There were times I asked others to read portions of what I had written and give me an evaluation of the content. I am especially grateful to those who took the time and effort to go beyond my questionnaire and write other helpful comments.

Teresa Hoffman was a good critic. She pasted helpful notes throughout the manuscript that gave encouragement and insight. She was also bold enough to say, "I don't know what you are trying to say." Other times she said that more information was needed.

Jenny Lee Mason, a past president of our lupus support group. corrected grammar and punctuation. That was a time-consuming task because of my deficiency in this area. She also suggested that I rearrange certain chapters.

My most faithful critic has been my patient wife, Beth. She dared to strain husband and wife relationships as she boldly challenged my thoughts and expressions. During our times of discussion about what I was writing, various thoughts would surface and she would say, "Why don't you write about it?"

Introduction

If someone had told me 15 years ago that I would be writing a book today, I'd have said, or at least thought, "You must be crazy! I can't write a book."

Writing is not my natural talent and, when it comes to grammar and spelling, I am probably the world's worst. It's difficult for me to get thoughts down on paper and make them flow. I'd rather talk to people face to face.

So why am I writing a book? During the past several years I have been challenged to do some writing because people have enjoyed hearing me tell about my various life experiences. I decided to write a small booklet, *Lupus Had Me Down,* to encourage other lupus patients. Some who read it have encouraged me to write a full-length book about my experiences, stating that nothing has been written by a male lupus patient. Since writing is not for me a natural or learned talent, there have been times when the writing came to a standstill. Then I would hear of someone who had been diagnosed as having lupus, or another chronic illness, and ask them to read what I had written. Their responses encouraged me to take up the pen once more.

Books are my friends. I often read portions of them time and again to find encouragement and help in what others have written. I consider reading to be part of the growing experience that is important to life. It is my hope that you will find portions of this book that you will choose to read more than once to help you when you are discouraged and need a lift to help you in your wilderness journey.

How did a disease get the name "lupus" and what does it mean? In the early days of diagnosing lupus, a doctor observed a rash across the nose of one patient and thought it gave the person a wolf- like appearance. "Lupus" is the Latin word for wolf and that is why the disease became known as "lupus."

Lupus is known to many as a woman's disease. I was very irritated when a doctor made that statement to me. My doctor had sold his practice, and the new doctor brought in several others to work with him. When I visited his office, I never knew which doctor I would see. On one visit the doctor who saw me stated, with a demeaning tone of voice, "Lupus is a woman's disease." I was aggravated at his callous remark and retorted, "Half of my ancestors are women; therefore, I have a right to have lupus, so don't try to deprive me of my rights." He then changed his comments by saying that very few men have lupus.

The phone rang one morning. When I answered it I realized that there was a very angry young man at the other end. He was in his late twenties and felt that he had been stripped of his manhood when he had been told he had lupus. He was unable to hold on to his job and, to make matters worse, well-meaning friends would say, "I thought that lupus was a woman's disease." He was not only emotionally disturbed by his illness, but the thought of having a "woman's disease" was almost more than he could bear.

I became vice president of our local lupus support group because others thought the group should have a male officer to encourage other male lupus patients. We have since had other male lupus patients attend the meetings and also serve on our board of directors.

Since then I have been president of the group and also started our regular newsletter to help keep people informed of our activities. My wife and I have also organized and conducted an annual lupus education seminar. We have been successful in enlisting other teachers and workers to help carry out the tasks of helping other lupus patients. Their lives as lupus patients have been enriched by their involvement in helping others.

The book is basically about living with a chronic illness. Mine happens to be lupus, but I have also included the experiences of others who are afflicted with multiple sclerosis, arthritis and chronic fatigue immune deficiency. Theirs are also chronic illnesses and they experience many of the same perplexing, emotional trials as lupus patients.

The thought of adventure is woven throughout the book as a challenge to the reader to look in new directions for hope and encouragement. To me, all of life is an adventure. An adventure brings zest to the routine, brightens the disagreeable and adverse situations, and even lifts the spirit to new heights during times of joy. My adventure began on a Kansas farm, took me to California and the south Pacific, and back to California. I will only pass through this life once, so why should I allow my chronic illness to spoil my adventure of living? I must make the illness itself part of that adventure.

When you are living through an adventure, at times you will experience uncomfortable, frightening, and unpleasant situations. That is part of the adventure; when it is over you may look back upon it with nostalgia.

My challenge is that you will see your illness from a new perspective and focus upon *life* and the adventure of living.

Chapter 1

Was It A Dream?

Savage wolves will come in among you and will not spare the flock.[1]

The wolf was slinking stealthily through the shadows, stalking its prey. Completely unaware of danger, I strode confidently through the forest. I had traveled this path before with no problem, so there was no reason to suspect trouble now. Suddenly the wolf sprang from the shadows, sinking his fangs in deeply. I trembled with fear and anger to be taken so completely by surprise. As I struggled to break away, I thought of shattered goals, disrupted schedules, and frustrated family. With every attempt to escape, I felt the fangs of the wolf again and again until I despaired of even life itself. "Why me? Why am I a victim of this creature?"

---

[1] Acts 20:29, New International Version

Although racked by pain and fever, I was able to momentarily escape the watchful eye of this predator. As I began to make my way out of the forest, I was pursued and brought down again and again. Was there no escape from this wild and fierce animal?

As I grew stronger and found nourishment, I was able to keep a little ahead of the wolf, though constantly aware of his presence. There were times when I thought I was escaping, only to hear the fearsome howl of the wolf echoing through the hills once again. Would I ever escape this wilderness where the wolf is at home and I am the stranger?

In some places the path was steep and full of obstacles that exhausted me as I made my way over the hills and through the valleys away from the ravaging wolf. However, as strength returned and escape seemed certain, the wolf would suddenly spring from the shadows and I felt those dreaded fangs once again. "Who am I, to be stalked night and day by this tenacious wolf?"

During the long wilderness journey, the wolf and I gained mutual respect. As I learned more of the wolf's ways and came to understand him in his natural environment, the journey became easier.

Did I finally escape the fierce wolf? How did I come to view this frightening attack in the lonely, hostile wilderness as an adventure?

Chapter 2

Just A Country Boy

Oh, I would that I were a boy again,
When life seemed formed of sunny years,
And all the heart then knew of pain
Was wept away in transient tears![1]

Growing up on a farm could be exciting for I was an adventurous, curious child who wanted to know how things worked. My clearest early childhood memories are focused on either a traumatic event or pain. I remember an incident that happened in 1922 when I was three years old.

My father was using block and tackle (pulleys and a rope) to pull hay up into the barn hayloft. I stood observing the rope pass through the pulleys with interest, but he had told me I must not touch it. So what did I do? I just *had* to feel it and as a result I have a finger that is still bent today.

---

[1] Mark Lemon, *Oh Would I Were a Boy Again*

Because I was the oldest boy of the family, my father gave me responsibilities that were not usually given to boys my age. It was an exciting time when he taught me to drive the tractor. When I was just six, my father would trust me with it and I would sit there like a king on a throne, driving through the field, while my father was busy with other farm work.

On a farm there are animals: horses, mules, cows, messy chickens, which I hated, and sometimes goats. When I was a young boy, the horses and mules didn't always want to obey me, so I had to use ingenuity.

Milking the cows was a routine morning and evening chore, and I can't remember when I started. I do have fond memories of our cats that would sit at the hind feet of the cow waiting for me to squirt milk in their mouths. It got to be more fun when I would squirt the milk over their faces and watch them lick it off.

We had two large beautiful mules that stood in marked contrast to our fine horses. I don't think a better team of mules could have been found anywhere. Mules have a very distinctive feature about them—they must be convinced who is boss! Occasionally my father had to do that by forcefully laying a two by four between their ears until they got the message. Even though I worked around them and with them, I was never able to convince them that I was the boss so we had a continuous battle.

My father had hitched the mules to the wagon so I could drive it to the field and gather hay. I was only six or seven at the time, and the mules decided not to obey and ran away with me. My father saw it and came racing through the field in the car. He gradually turned the mules toward a barbed wire fence and stopped them at the corner of the field. After literally pounding some sense into their heads, he drove the team back to the corral, and I drove the car.

There was one more traumatic confrontation with those stubborn mules. I had gone to the barn to feed the horses and mules, which were in their stalls waiting for food. I threw some hay down from the hay loft. Then I would take a pitchfork of hay, call the animal by name and say "move over." The horses usually moved over so that, approaching from behind, I could go between them and their stall. Everything was proceeding without problems until I came to the mules. I would approach the mule from one side; he would move to block me and look at me with those demon eyes. I would try the other side, and he would move to block me again; I could see the hatred in his eye. I became angry, dropped the hay, jabbed him in the hindquarter with the pitch fork, and saw his hind foot coming at me. When I woke up, I was lying in a pool of blood a good distance from the mule.

My mother almost fainted when I walked into the kitchen with a large gash in my head, covered with blood. At the hospital the doctor said he wanted to put me to sleep before cleaning and suturing the wound. He asked my mother; "Has he had anything to eat recently?" She said, "No, we haven't had supper yet." My mother later told me that after the anesthetic had put me under, I vomited corn, vegetables and melons all over the table and the surrounding floor. Down on the farm we didn't go to the cookie jar when we were hungry; we went to the garden and ate what we wanted!

My episodes with the mules proved the reality of a little jingle we used to sing:

"Get along, mule, don't you roll them eyes!
You can change a fool but a dog-gone mule
Is a mule until he dies."

Harvest was an exciting time. Each summer my father hired a school teacher to help with the harvest. He was usually paid the large sum of one dollar per day plus room and board. The new hired hand was more than just a worker—he was a teacher, a person of dignity. We considered it an honor to have a teacher living with us. Sometimes we rode on the wagon with him as he took the wheat to market. He told us adventurous stories that appealed to our imaginations. He also told us interesting things about the school where he was teaching.

The last day of harvest was a festive occasion. My father bought a five gallon can of ice cream and we would gather under the large cottonwood tree for a "store boughten" ice cream feast. Those were the "good ol' days." Now home-made ice cream is a treat.

We moved from St. John, Kansas, to Springfield, Colorado, when I was eleven years old. The years on the farm in Colorado were also adventurous years. We got together with neighbors for our own rodeos. We rode bucking steers bareback with nothing to hang on to; there was steer roping, bull dogging, horse racing, and whatever else we could think up.

The strawberry roan horse was my favorite for working cattle. One day when I wanted him, he was out in the pasture. I got on another horse to bring him in so I could bridle and saddle him. As we approached the strawberry roan, he reared up on his hind legs with his front hooves flailing the air as he tried to knock me off the horse I was riding. I went back to the house, got my rifle, and went after the strawberry roan once again. He saw the rifle, laid his ears back, and headed for the corral without any more trouble.

The Midwest is often referred to as the "bible-belt." Our family attended Sunday school and church every Sunday. Kids can be ornery even when they are in church. I recall the evening when I sneaked out of church, went to the movie theater, sneaked in and sat in the front row. Before I got engrossed in the movie, I was looking straight into the barrel of a gun. It was on the screen; however, the appearance was so real that I fled the theater and sneaked back into church. That was my first experience of going to the movies.

I enjoyed sports, playing football and basketball and also participating in track meets. In basketball I always played center; I can't remember anyone who could jump higher than I could. That gave our team a little edge over the others. In track meets I always won the high jumping and broad jumping contests with very little effort.

Through a tragic accident, my father perished in a fire, and my mother was left with seven children to raise. A year later, when I was sixteen, my younger brother and I went to California to live with an uncle.

The train ride from Lamar, Colorado, to Pasadena, California, was a great adventure. We climbed up through the Rocky Mountains and eventually were speeding through the wide open spaces. Though all the scenery was spellbinding, I had an abundance of energy to work off and a curiosity to be satisfied, so I began to explore the train.

I discovered that the car next to mine was filled with a wild bunch of young men who had joined the Navy and were on their way to boot camp at San Diego, California. They were enthusiastic, energetic, and active. I enjoyed their company and spent a lot of my time in their car.

As we were approaching the Pasadena area, I was captivated by the sight of so many orange trees. As we passed through mile after mile of orange groves, I wondered who was going to eat all of those oranges. On our farm in Colorado, we didn't even have a fruit tree.

The conductor announced that we had arrived at Pasadena. My aunt and a cousin were waiting for us, and we were soon driving along Colorado Boulevard. I found it amazing that it was the main street of Pasadena since I couldn't see either end of the street! Never had I seen a city that large.

I soon found a job squeezing orange juice. After I received my first pay check, my aunt wanted room and board money. She firmly declared, "Everyone must pay his own way."

Before the year was over, I had found a job driving a dump truck if I could obtain a chauffeur's license. I lied about my age and got the license; from that day on I was in a man's world. As a truck driver I worked on numerous construction jobs, mostly road construction.

One job that I have fond memories of was on Towne Pass between Death Valley and Panamint Valley. We camped in tents at a settlement (a couple of houses, a service station, and a cafe) called Panamint Springs. Our favorite place to take a shower was two or three miles away at Darwin Waterfalls. The water just ran out of the ground over a rocky cliff and disappeared again in a short distance. Forty years later, my wife and I were traveling through that area and I said, "I wonder if I can find the waterfall." There were no signs to tell where it was, but after thinking for a while and a little exploring we found a trickle of water and followed it to the fall.

There were other road construction jobs in the San Joaquin Valley and also near San Diego. The work was adventurous because we would usually stay in one place for a few months and had the opportunity to get acquainted with many of the people in the area. I soon had friends from San Diego to San Francisco.

When construction work slowed down, I went to work in a foundry. That was hard work; at times I was swinging a forty-two pound (not a misprint) sledge hammer smashing a worn-out engine block with one blow. I would then load a thousand pounds of scrap iron on a cart and push it into the foundry to be melted for castings.

Even though the work was hard, I took it in stride to support my first love—motorcycles. Auto and motorcycle racing had captivated my interest and would soon have a powerful influence upon me. I had several friends who raced autos; however, I was too tall to get into the race cars they had in those days so I decided that I would race motorcycles.

At that time, 1940, there was lots of talk about the possibility of war. The draft board was threatening every able-bodied young man who was not employed in defense work so I got a job in a San Francisco shipyard foundry. We cast many valves and other parts, including nine and one-half ton propellers for the destroyers they were building.

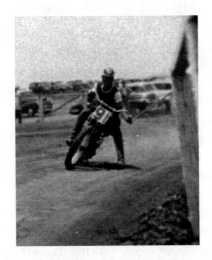

On the half mile flat track.

Despite the war talk and need for being employed in defense work for deferment from the draft, a friend and I were planning a tour across country doing nothing but racing motorcycles. Our goal was first and second place in each race; we also had our sights set upon the two-hundred mile national championship race at Daytona Beach, Florida. However, those plans were put on hold because of World War II.

Defense work was no longer a deferment from the draft, and I was ordered to report for a physical examination. At the conclusion, the doctor looked me in the eye and said, "Disgustingly healthy." I knew that meant that I would soon be inducted into the Army. The next day I volunteered for the Navy.

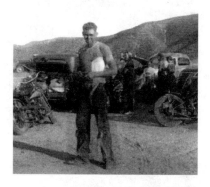

After a grueling desert race.
My motorcycle is the one on the left.

The physical examination for the Navy was different from that of the Army. They gave more attention to smaller details. When a doctor noticed my bent finger, he extended his hand and said, "Take hold of my hand and squeeze." I had a vice-like grip, and when I squeezed, he let out a yell. The old saying that misery loves company came into play. He sent me to another doctor, calling attention to my bent finger. The other doctor was a little more cautious, he held out a finger and said, "Take hold of my finger and pull." I jerked him out of his chair, and he decided that my bent finger was not a problem.

Just a few days later I was sworn into the Navy. A day or two after that I was notified by the draft board to report on a certain day and be sworn into the Army. I reported but told them that they were too late, I was already in the Navy—a move I have never regretted.

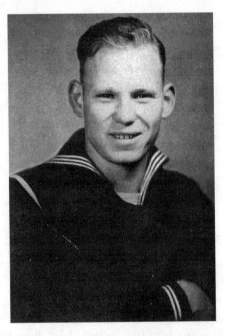

Life of Ol' Salt. Many complained about their military service. To me, it was an adventure that has left me with memories that I will continue to cherish.

Chapter 3

World War II

The quiet words of the wise are more to be heeded
than the shouts of a ruler of fools. Wisdom is better
than the weapons of war.[1]

My first sea duty was aboard the seagoing tug
Bobolink. I went aboard her in Pearl Harbor and
three days later we set sail for New Caledonia, then
to the New Hebrides and finally Guadalcanal in the
South Pacific. The Guadalcanal campaign was
harder on the Navy than any other Pacific battle.[2]
There were so many ships resting on the bottom of
the bay between Guadalcanal, Tulaghi, and Savo
Islands that we referred to it as *Iron Bottom Bay*.
We were the first seagoing tug that lasted more
than three days.

---

[1] Ecclesiastes 9:17-18, New International Version

[2] United States Naval Institute, *United States Destroyer Operations in World War II*, Chapter 15

On our third day, we had quite a scare. It was just after daybreak, and the water surface was glassy smooth. The decks of our ship were loaded with fifty gallon drums of aviation gasoline and five hundred pound bombs. We were also towing a large barge loaded with the same type cargo. Another crew member and I were standing on deck when we suddenly saw what appeared to be a submarine periscope, and it started moving directly toward us. We looked at one another and headed for our battle stations. About that time, someone on the bridge saw the same thing and sounded general quarters. The periscope turned out to be only the dorsal fin of a shark. Nevertheless, we were apprehensive until that third day had passed.

Our ship was not considered a fighting vessel, although we were credited with sinking a Japanese submarine. We were making our way across the channel from Tulaghi to Guadalcanal when a submarine stuck its periscope up just astern of us. We dropped a couple of depth charges and shortly afterwards enough debris surfaced to satisfy us that we got him.

We were often called upon to tow damaged ships out of the battle area and one time were being fired upon by the Japanese battleship *Hiei*. The battleship was silenced by land-based dive bombers.

We also assisted ships that had been torpedoed and were on fire; their crews were abandoning ship on one side, and we would board it on the other, fighting the fire and eventually towing the ship to safety so that it could be temporarily repaired and able to sail for home port.

We worked two days and one night with one ship. The ship had fifty gallon drums of aviation gasoline in the forward cargo hold and every time one would explode it would lift us off the deck a few inches. After getting the fire under control, we finally beached the ship on the coast of Guadalcanal, and there it stayed until it could be repaired enough to float once again.

Other times we would go into the battle area and tow away damaged ships. Some of the sights we saw will be with me as long as I live. I remember a once proud cruiser, *USS Atlanta*, punched full of shell holes, with charred bodies draped over the lifeline. She was riding so low in the water we knew that all hands below deck would never see the light of day again. Another time we saw a mighty warrior with its bow blown off and a large portion of her crew sealed in a watery grave. It was almost hard to understand that a ship could be there one moment and gone an instant later.

The *USS Portland* had taken a torpedo in the stern section that jammed the rudder so that it could only go in circles. At the end of the day, we were helping it back to Tulaghi Harbor. Nightfall had overtaken us. The PT boats were heading out for their night patrol and were told that all of our ships were in. When they spotted us, they launched a volley of torpedoes toward us. Because of the way that our ship and the *Portland* were working together, we made a large wake, and those aboard the PT boats miscalculated our speed, and the torpedoes passed well ahead of us. The skipper of the Portland called saying, "Bobolink! Bobolink! Talk to those PT boasts. My whole naval career depends on you!" We radioed the PT boats, and they called off their attack.

The next morning we saw a sight that most people will never see. Tulaghi Harbor was not very large, and there were two damaged ships that were tied fore and aft to coconut trees. We did have another unusual happening. We had to tow a PT boat out of the jungle. The Japanese learned that their destroyers could out-run the PT boats. One evening a destroyer went through the smoke screen heading for the PT boat. The PT boat headed for the beach and went all the way into the jungle. I guess that is one way to hide a large boat. In this case it was more effective than the smoke screen.

After a year on the *Bobolink* and a year of shore patrol duty in the war zone, I was sent back to San Francisco and eventually placed in a destroyer pool awaiting ship assignment.

Coming back to civilization was a miserable experience. So many things had changed and most of my friends were in the military service. I didn't seem to fit in anywhere and I wanted to go back to the war zone. About the only good thing that happened during that thirty days was that I met a pretty nurse who would later become my wife. She will tell the story of it in a later chapter.

While I was on liberty, in Oakland, California, I stepped into a hospitality house for servicemen. I sat on a couch and noticed a New Testament on the table. I picked it up and saw that several pages had the corners turned down pointing to 1 John 5:4 where I read: "For everyone born of God overcomes the world. This is the victory that overcomes the world, even our faith. Who is it that overcomes the world? Only he who believes that Jesus is the Son of God."

Those verses spoke about *victory* and *overcoming the world;* that was what I felt that I needed more than anything else. I read the two verses over and over and discovered that I had memorized them.

On one of my liberties, I went to a Servicemen's Center in the basement of the College Avenue Presbyterian Church in Oakland, California. The place was alive with wholesome activities— something I was not used to. I decided that I would attend church service the next Sunday morning and that morning I committed my life to Jesus as my Lord and Savior.

As I strolled through a park that afternoon and heard the birds responding with hearty song to the balmy fall weather, it seemed they were putting on a performance just for me. The flowers were beautiful and looked very delicate. Everything was alive, and I felt in tune with nature. Though I went to the park alone, it seemed that I never met a stranger. I made conversation with a number of different people, old and young alike. When we parted company, it was as though we had just renewed an old acquaintance. That day was certainly a new beginning for me and also the beginning of a new life-long adventure. I no longer wanted to go back to the war zone, but knew that was where I would be sent.

Shortly after this I was sent to Bremerton, Washington to board my new assignment, the destroyer, *USS Zellars.* The shipyard workers were still putting the finishing touches on it when we arrived.

I was assigned to the after engine room and, although everything was different from the tug, I loved it! Over the next several weeks I worked hard to learn all I could about the engine room and its operation. The day finally came for our first test cruise. I never left the engine room during that one-day cruise. That was *my* place and I felt that that was where I belonged!

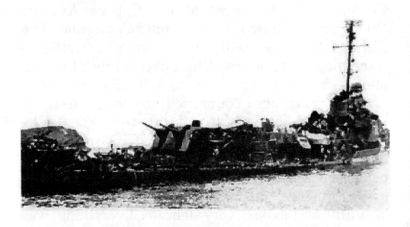

The minelayer *Aaron Ward* after being blasted by kamikazes while in the company with *Little*, which sank at Okinawa with fourteen other destroyers and destroyer-escorts

While we were at the Bremerton shipyards, a destroyer returned from the war zone. It had been hit by several suicide planes, and most of its superstructure was flattened almost to the deck. As I stood on the dock and looked at it, particularly at the area where I had been assigned for battle duty, I thought, "If I had been aboard that ship, I wouldn't be here today."

That was a sobering sight and thought! As I stood there looking at it, in a most unusual manner God assured me that I would not suffer any harm in battle while aboard my ship. Don't ask me to explain that! It was one of those rare moments a person may have in his walk with God.

After the shake-down cruise, we were sent to Hawaii for operations training with other ships. This included all kinds of gunnery practice, simulated damage control, and all of the other things that may occur in battle.

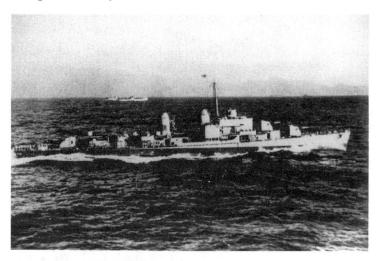

USS *Zellars* off the Coast of Hawaii

While we were in Hawaii, I wanted to find Christian friends. One evening, while I was lying on the fantail of the ship and looking up at the stars, I was also asking the Lord what I should do to find others who knew Him so that I might be encouraged in my new Christian life. The answer seemed to be, "Why don't you start a Bible class?"

"Who? Me? I don't know anything about the Bible. How can I start a Bible class?"

"I didn't ask you how much you knew. I have only asked you to start a Bible class. I will teach you," was the Lord's reply.

I told the Lord that I didn't even have a complete Bible and the answer was "Go over on the beach and buy one," which I did a few days later.

I got up from the deck and spoke to the first person I saw about starting a Bible class. He told me that one of the men who had come aboard two days before wanted to start church services. I found that man, and as we talked, he asked me to help him with church services. I told him that God wanted me to start a Bible class. He said, "Let's help each other." This gave new dimension to the adventure that I had already embarked upon, an adventure that was exciting and filled with life!

In a few weeks we were part of the great armada of ships (the largest in naval history) leaving the Caroline Islands and bound for Okinawa. Okinawa was the last island we needed to conquer before making an assault upon the Japanese mainland. The war had taken its toll on the Imperial Navy and most of Japan's ships were lying on the ocean floor. However, there was one last barbaric effort lurking in the dark shadows of the war, especially for destroyers—the kamikaze (Divine Wind). Naval books attest to the fact that in all of the war, no ships ever had to fight so hard or suffer so much loss of life and ship as the destroyers did at Okinawa in Japan's suicidal assault.

Our ship was one of the casualties. There were three kamikazes that made their run upon us. Only one plane and the engine of another hit us, but that was all that it took to put us out of action. My battle duties were mid-ship damage control. I had just arrived at my station and was putting on my helmet when we were hit. The ship lunged to starboard, then reeled back to port side as the bomb exploded. My helmet was blown from my hands. I saw fire on both sides of the mid-ship passageway. Dead bodies were lying on the decks and a good friend was killed at my side.

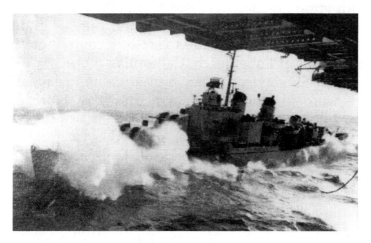

USS *Zellars* fueling at sea in the South Pacific near the international dateline.

I grabbed a fire hose and headed into the fire. Flames were all around me. The 40 millimeter ammunition locker, directly above me, could explode at any moment. I opened the valve to flood it with water. Voices called out, "Help us! Help us down here!" Shipmates were trapped below deck. There was a blazing inferno above them. I was there in the middle of it. Abruptly my fire hose went dead. There I stood with fire all around me. Suddenly I felt cold water; a solid stream of high pressure water was trained on me. He should have been using a spray; however, what he was doing probably saved me from severe burns.

Through all of that, I never received the slightest injury, not even a singed hair. God had kept His promise to me. The ones who were calling for help were rescued. Our ship had a crew of three hundred forty-five and we suffered seventy-five casualties with approximately half of them killed.

After making temporary repairs, our wounded ship and crew were ready to set our course for the ship yards at Long Beach, California.

It was Sunday morning, a bright sunny day, and we were to leave for home the next morning. General quarters sounded; we were under attack by a kamikaze. The crew was gripped by fear. Many were hanging on the outside of the ship's lifeline ready to dive into the water at any moment, and most of our guns couldn't fire. The kamikaze hit another ship; the threat to us was over. The ship's speaker system blared out, "Secure from General Quarters", and a moment later, "Church services will be conducted in the crew's mess [hall]." I was still trembling from the threat of our ship being hit once again, and now I was also scared half to death because I was to be the speaker (my first time) at the church service. Fear motivated many of the crew to attend the service. The place was jam-packed, and I learned later that many were unable to get in. I don't remember what I had to say that day, but I can remember that for the next several days there was a noticeable lack of swearing and foul language. We were all affected by deep gratitude to God that we were spared further loss of life and injury.

The ship wasn't even one year old, and we were out of action. However, during that time we had shot down several suicide planes, shelled the beach in preparation for troops to land, and were in a decoy force to draw fire away from the troop landing. We also gave fire support for the ground forces and were among the ships that went after the remainder of the Japanese Navy, which included their prize battleship, *Yamato*, with her awesome eighteen-inch guns.

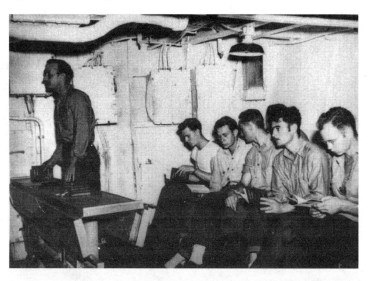

Chapel Services aboard the ship. I am on the extreme right. The one standing started the chapel services.

On the way home as we were entering Pearl Harbor for fuel and supplies, I saw the *Bobolink*. I had the signalmen contact her, and later in the day I enjoyed a nice reunion with some of my former shipmates. They enjoyed their visit to my ship as I showed them through it and explained the battles we had been through and the resulting damage.

I had been at sea for ninety days without setting foot on land when we sailed into Long Beach,

California and tied up to a wharf. A large container of ice cream bars and cartons of milk were placed on deck. Photographers and news reporters swarmed aboard. My mother, brother (who was not in the service due to a physical handicap), youngest sister and sister-in-law (who were living in Pasadena) had not heard from me for more than three months when Sunday morning they saw my picture on the front page of the *Herald Examiner*. There I was, standing on the deck of a mangled ship, drinking a quart of milk. The paper said that visitors were welcome, and that afternoon I had the pleasure of showing them through the ship. I told them about the battles and explained the damage we received.

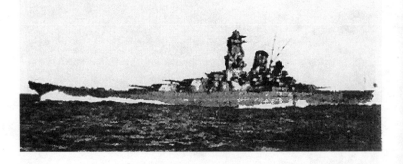

The *Yamato*

Repairs were made and shortly after another shake-down cruise, the war was over. It was not long until I received the news that I was eligible for discharge. It was a happy day when I received my discharge papers and was a civilian once more.

Chapter 4

Me, Chronically Ill?

What I feared has come upon me;
what I dreaded has happened to me.
I have no peace, no quietness;
I have no rest, but only turmoil.[1]

Since my life had new orientation after committing it to Jesus as Lord, I was aware that I needed more education. It took me three days to complete the GED test to receive my high school diploma and then on to the Bible Institute of Los Angeles (BIOLA) for the next four years. After my first year at BIOLA I married Beth Baker, the charming nurse I met during the war. She was born and raised among the orange groves near Fillmore, California. Sometimes I affectionately call her my "orange blossom." Before I graduated we had our first child—a beautiful daughter, Audrey.

---

[1] Job 3:25-26, New International Version

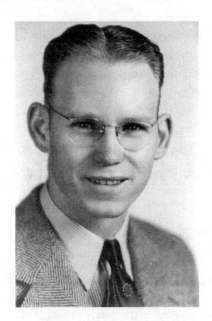

Robert's Senior Picture

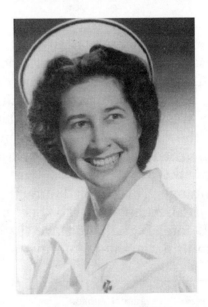

Beth's Senior Picture

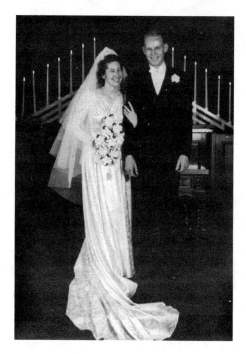

Wedding Photo

After graduation, I spent the next twenty years starting new churches. I have always had boundless energy and have enthusiastically accepted new challenges, which filled those years. By the time I was approaching fifty years of age and most of the churches were looking for younger men, I found it necessary to search for a new career. Those who thought I was too old should have listened to my daughter. She told some of her school friends that "My daddy will never be in his second childhood—he's never going to get out of his first one."

Snap-On Tools did not see me as being too old to be a good salesman. I often won "Top Salesman" of the year award and many other sales contest awards during my thirteen years with the company.

While I was at the very height of my earning power (my income was a percentage of what I sold), I realized that something was wrong with me. My legs were stiff and my left leg would get completely numb. My neck became stiff, and it was painful to turn my head. I was experiencing extreme fatigue and finding it difficult to keep up with my daily tasks. Finally I was running a fever of 102 degrees every afternoon.

Out-patient tests became the routine for the next several weeks. After the ordeal of a barium enema, I staggered down the hall like a drunken man, bouncing from wall to wall. I had been getting progressively weaker, and the barium enema was almost the final blow to what strength I had.

Finally, I was placed in the hospital for more tests. In spite of the fact that I didn't like hospitals, the next two weeks turned out to be an interesting adventure. I was assigned to a team of doctors and being involved with them added interest to the days. When I was taken to the nuclear department for tests, I recognized some of the equipment since I had been selling tools to the company that built the machines.

Later, an expectorant test was ordered and that turned out to be rather hilarious. A rather timid nurse brought in a plastic bag and said, "We need an expectorant sample from you," hung the bag on the bed, and left the room.

Since I couldn't cough up a sample, they sent in an aggressive nurse to beat it out of me! She came in with a whole battery of equipment and the determination of a military drill sergeant to make me perform. She placed a mask over my face, turned on the fumigation gas and commanded, "Breathe deeply." After taking off the mask, she held out a plastic bag and commanded, "Cough!" After a couple of repeated efforts, she commanded, "Roll over!" She then placed a pillow under my chest and the mask on my face for another round that took me by surprise. "Breathe deep. Breathe some more." Then she jumped on top of me and began pounding my back with both of her fists and shouting, "Cough! Cough! Cough!" I began to laugh so hard that she finally gave up. She then said, "I'll bet you'll be glad when this mean ol' nurse is gone."

"No! This is the most fun I have had since I got sick," I replied.

That episode kind of got my ornery nature going again so I began to play tricks on the nurses and other hospital personnel just to help put a little humor into the routine. It didn't help the diagnosis, but it did help me to feel better.

They had just about run out of tests to give me when X-rays revealed a spot on one of my lungs. Since they couldn't get an expectorant test from me, a lung specialist was called in. He had read all of the reports, examined the X-rays, then came to my room and began to ask questions. I told him of the symptoms that I thought the doctors should have been more concerned about. I told him that before becoming ill I had been running a mile and a half every other morning with ease and intended to work up to two miles. But, it became painful so I cut back to a mile, then a half mile, and finally quit because running even a half mile was painful. I told him that my neck was extremely stiff, especially turning it to the left, and about the numb feeling in my left leg. I also told him that I could no longer ride any distance on my motorcycle. He asked me many more questions and finally stated that the spot on my lung was nothing but scar tissue and that he would not discount lupus being my problem.

I told him that since my mother had lupus I had been tested for it, and the results were negative. He said, "I wouldn't rely upon one test; they should test several times." Once again the crew returned to draw more blood. I thought, "Will this never end? How much more blood are they going to draw from me?" The doctors had told me that I was anemic and I asked, "What can you expect since the vampires have drawn so much blood for all those tests?"

After two weeks of testing, I was sent home without a diagnosis. By now I had been in bed for more than two months and felt very sick. The late November weather was almost like summer, and I asked my wife, "Would you buy me a patio chaise lounge? I am going to lie in the sunshine and bake this thing out of me." Later I learned that for some lupus patients that is exactly the wrong treatment.

I continued to get worse and also became deeply depressed. I had expected the doctors to find out what was wrong with me and get me back to normal. All of the testing, doctors' efforts, and everything else seemed to be a total failure so I concluded that death was better than life. I had surrendered all hope and reached the stage that I would not hesitate to take my own life. When I said so, my wife almost went into shock. As I think back upon that time, it is also shocking to me that the once healthy, energetic, athletic, competitive person would give up so easily.

A few days after the onset of depression, my doctor called and said, "The latest tests indicate that you probably have lupus." He prescribed 40 milligrams of prednisone morning and evening. I took my first dose that afternoon, unprepared for its effect upon me. The next morning the depression was gone and I felt great! I could kick higher than my head, something I hadn't done since my football days in high school. I was feeling so great that after breakfast I wanted to take a brisk walk around the block. I hadn't gone a half-block when I knew that I should return home while I had the strength to make it back.

I was now faced with a new problem: "How am I going to live with this?" My wife is a registered nurse and the two of us set out to learn all we could about lupus. The hospital tape recording said, "Systemic Lupus Erythematosus (SLE) is a chronic illness, and there is no known cure. Life expectancy is five years." That was in 1981, and the short life expectancy is no longer true. However, it is a chronic condition that I had to learn to live with.

My doctor started me out on 80 milligrams of prednisone a day which is a very large dosage. He told me to reduce the dosage each week to 60 milligrams, 40 milligrams, 20 milligrams, then after a week go back to work. When I got down to 40 milligrams per day, I called him and said that I couldn't get along on the smaller dosage. He said that he wanted me off it as quickly as possible because he didn't like the potential side effects. I told him that I would rather chance the side effects than to have the ill feeling all of the time. He told me to continue taking 60 milligrams a day for a while.[2]

I didn't go back to work for another month, and then I worked only half-days for several months. That tired and weak feeling was persistently with me. I felt that life would never be the same again.

I was a man who for more than sixty years had been "disgustingly healthy," who avoided people who were ill or handicapped, and had now been cut down. Would I be a victim of this chronic illness, or would I see it as a challenge to *live*? Would I just learn to cope with my illness, or turn it into another adventure?

---

[2] The doctor gradually worked me down to 15 milligrams a day and later to 15 milligrams every other day which I took for at least two years. I eventually was on and off prednisone as the flares and remissions would come and go.

Chapter 5

My Illness, an Adventure?

Adventure embraces joy, exhilaration, discouragement, danger, times of easy going and adversity.

How can anyone think of a chronic illness as an adventure? I have always thought of an adventure as being enjoyable and exciting. I don't see how this can apply to me now that I have a chronic illness. Won't I also be a chronic complainer? How can I look upon my condition as an adventure? This is not something I wanted. If it is an adventure, I want out!

Emotions and feelings can become quite turbulent when a person is challenged to look at his or her life-threatening illness from a viewpoint other than fear, anger, or self-pity. However, that is the challenge of this book, to help you to see your situation from a new viewpoint. It is my hope that you will find encouragement through it.

The thought of turning my own illness into an adventure came to me in the early days of my encounter with lupus. Several years prior to my illness, I had read a book, *The Adventure of Living*, by Dr. Paul Tournier. I remembered that the last portion of the book was written after his own illness. He wrote from the perspective that life would never be the same for him, and he had to adjust to it. As I read the book once again, I was challenged by the idea that I must learn to live within my own natural environment. My body *is* my natural environment; therefore, my illness must become a part of my adventure in life.

For an illustration, we can think of our astronauts. In this space age we have sent men to the moon where they were in a totally different environment. The astronauts were limited in their activities on the moon because they had to move within the environment they took with them. Their bulky space suits carried their own oxygen supply, temperature control, communication equipment, and everything else that was needed for them to live on the surface of the moon. Despite their limitations, their experience was a great adventure. While we joined their adventure through our television sets, it was not the same as theirs.

The thought of turning your illness into an adventure may be hard to handle, especially if you have been healthy and active. However, the key thoughts are *learn* and *live*, just as the astronauts had to train and learn how to live a short while on the surface of the moon. Your life has a new dimension added to it, and you must now *learn* to *live* in an environment that seems foreign, and possibly hostile.

Writing this book was a new adventure that had been interrupted because of the necessity of hand surgery. Dupuytren's Contracture was causing my fingers to curl in towards the palm of my hand so I could no longer work at my computer without putting in all kinds of letters that didn't belong there. While I was without the use of my right hand following surgery, I decided to turn it into an adventure and live as a one-armed man.

Among the numerous things I discovered about life for a man with only one arm was that the simple things of life became complicated and awkward. I will mention only a few of them.

Before I left the hospital, I had to change from the surgery garments to my street clothing. I was struggling to put on my socks with only my left hand. My wife wanted to help, but I said that I might just as well start doing it myself. Since then I have told others about how difficult it is to put socks on with only a left hand. It has been amusing to hear so many tell me that they have tried it and finally given up. There is a difference when you have only one hand to use—you have to succeed.

I needed to wash and dry my left hand. Did you ever try to scrub your hand with the only hand you have? Then drying it on a towel was another source of aggravation. I finally gave up with the towel and used the best method I knew—there is no substitute for a pants leg!

Breakfast also created new problems. I sometimes enjoy a slice of toast with honey for breakfast. Fall weather was setting in and because of the cooler temperatures, the honey in the jar was stiff. After a long struggle to take the lid off the jar and then scoop out a spoonful of honey, I faced the problem of getting the honey off the spoon and spreading it on the toast. It was no trouble scraping the honey off the back of the spoon onto the toast. When I turned the spoon over I had a major problem— getting the honey off the spoon. After some struggle, I managed to get the honey on the toast. When I tried to spread it, the toast would not hold still. I chased it all over the plate for a while and finally ate the toast without spreading the honey from edge to edge.

Now if you think that experience is humorous or tough, what would it be for a person with no hands? I recalled a time when I was attending an out-of-town business meeting. A group of us went to lunch, including one man who had only steel hooks for hands. He ordered a hamburger. This was in the days before McDonalds, and a hamburger was considerably larger than those of the fast food places today. When the hamburger was placed before him, I wondered if his wife would have to feed it to him. To my amazement, I saw the steel hook on one arm spread apart as he scooped up the hamburger and handled it in style. Later, he took a pen from his pocket to make notes of our conversation. His penmanship was far better than mine. Now I am sure that he would have preferred two hands to the steel hooks, and I am also sure that his wife would have preferred the touch of a warm hand to that of cold steel. Neither of them was complaining. They had adjusted to their new environment and were making the best of it. Any of us who are handicapped need to creatively turn the handicap or infirmity into an adventure.

As a result of my hand surgery, I have learned more about adventure through the process of my experiment. Adventure is one of our needs in life so that we may escape drab routine and restore our spirits. When we turn a misfortune into an adventure, that helps to remove the self-pity and other negative emotions that may overwhelm us. It is far more satisfying than hiding behind the infirmity. This type of adventure must emphasize the *quality* of life. We must distinguish between *quality* and *quantity*. Quantity is the seeking of many things: money, clothing, cars, entertainment, and an abundance of activities. We can never get enough to satisfy our appetites and we must remember that life does not consist in the abundance of things. On the other hand, quality is that of appreciating the finer side of life that *things* can never satisfy.

As I look back upon my seventy-five years of life, that which has brought the most satisfying quality to life has come through disappointments, struggles, the tough battles of World War II, and even my illness. I also remember the numerous times of joy, fun and pleasurable experiences. We need the balance; however the trials of life build strong character.

Let me illustrate this thought by referring to some remodeling that I needed to do on my house. To accomplish what I wanted, I used heavy timbers to build a supporting framework. The walls, windows and door have nothing to do with structural strength. They were placed there for my comfort and appreciation. Long ago I had learned that the struggles of life become the strong supporting framework, and the pleasant times are for my comfort and enjoyment. When I endeavor to comfort others in need, it is never accomplished through relating the good times that I have had in life, but only by relating the struggles and adversities of life. I ran across a poem by an unknown author that is apropos:

> I walked a mile with Pleasure,
> She chatted all the way,
> But left me none the wiser
> For all she had to say.

> I walked a mile with Sorrow,
> And ne'r a word said she,
> But, oh, the things I learned from her
> When Sorrow walked with me.

It is our conflicts, struggles, and suffering that bring depth and quality to the adventure of living.

If good times and pleasure were the essence of life, then life would have very little meaning. The good times and pleasures can be swept away rather quickly, as some of us are experiencing. I have learned to appreciate the fact that there is more to life than seeking pleasure, comfort, and all of the things that are commonly referred to as "the good life."

In an illness, adventure begins when we find creative ways to live with it and then use what we have discovered to help others. This requires commitment, and commitment requires putting down new roots. Probably the first question that should be resolved is: Am I going to pay the price for quality adventure? Adventures can become dull and fade away. For the chronically ill, who are seeking quality of life, there must be a commitment to keeping the adventure alive.

My adventure has been kept alive by my commitment to help and encourage others. Though I no longer feel the need for a support group, I like to attend so that I can aid others in need. This has led to speaking opportunities, radio and television appearances, writing articles and now a book. Before I became ill, I never dreamed that this would be a part of my life adventure.

I also discovered that there are many good things that keep us from the adventure. My writing schedule was interrupted by the need to remodel my house and then to have hand surgery. Through these interruptions, I discovered that a new commitment was necessary. Long before New Year's Day (New Year's resolutions are soon broken), I made a resolution that starting January 2, 1990, I was going to work four hours per day, five days per week until I finished the manuscript. I knew that before the manuscript was completed many good things would battle for the time that I wanted for writing.

Hindrances must either be swept aside or become part of the adventure. While I was laid up with hand surgery, I continued to do background reading and used a tape recorder for note taking and then— just let my imagination run wild. Adventure is only found in the dynamic movement of life; my recovery from surgery became a part of the adventure. One unexpected benefit is that I have enjoyed my left hand so much that I often hear the remark, "I didn't know that you were left-handed."

This book embraces personal experiences of people living with a chronic illness: two with multiple sclerosis, another with severe arthritis, and my own encounter with lupus.

I am very much aware that there are many other chronic conditions that others must live with and they need to hear from someone who is living with the same illness. I wish I could write about all of them; however, that is not the intent of this book. Regardless of what may be the cause of your suffering, we all have one common denominator: We have to live with it, and how we do so is of vital concern.

Many times I have talked to people who wonder how they can make it from one day to the next. I have seen the effect of their illnesses upon their bodies, and I know that they often wonder if they will ever "have a nice day." If this describes your condition, I can imagine your puzzlement as you read the title of this book and tried to imagine your illness as being an adventure in life.

I also know that the spectrum of a chronic condition ranges from mild to physically debilitating and life threatening. My own condition is considered mild, although three months in bed at three different times did not seem mild. I wish to be sensitive to your needs and hope that I do not discourage anyone. I would not want to create in anyone the feeling that there must be something wrong with you if you cannot see your situation as an adventure in life. However, it is my hope that you may be challenged to view your condition with an attitude that will allow you the freedom to live within your situation, rather than to feel that you are a victim of it.

There is one exercise we can all do when we are feeling sorry for ourselves and wondering "Why is this happening to me?" Just look around and see someone whose condition is worse than yours. Kay, a friend of mine, had always been healthy and active. Though it was unforeseen, she had blood clots lodge in her feet that resulted in bilateral amputation. Now that was a sudden and drastic turn of events! After surgery, she entered physical therapy, which was conducted in a group setting. During therapy she saw several others whose conditions were worse than her own. Kay said, "I am thankful that I have only lost my feet." When I heard that, I knew that she had won her battle. No, she will never have her own two feet again, but she is not defeated in her situation. With a gleam in her eyes she said, "When I get my prosthesis, I won't have so much trouble finding shoes that fit my small feet. They will be made to a standard size."

Finding ways to encourage others is good therapy. When I was struck with my second devastating three-month flare of lupus, I called to encourage a couple of other lupus patients. As we talked, I guessed they thought I was the one who needed cheering. They must have been thinking, "That poor guy, why is he trying to comfort me when he sounds like he may have one foot in the grave?" I shall never forget the tender tone of their voices as they endeavored to give me a lift. I could feel their empathy as they spoke. I was trying to help them, but I was the one who was being helped. That was a precious part of my adventure that I will always hold dear. This is also the adventure you will discover through attending a support group. Try it! It will do you good!

I would like to challenge you, if you are depressed and wondering if you will ever see a bright day again, to look around you and to look up for hope and encouragement. I know that it is difficult not to focus on how miserable you feel, but a change of focus may be the very thing that is needed to give you a lift, new insight and new hope. Norman Cousins in his book, *Head First* , has demonstrated that focusing our minds on the positive emotions (love, hope, faith, will to live, festivity, purpose, determination[1]) can actually reduce pain.

While I was attending a writers conference, I heard a man pray, "We are on a journey through life. The soul that is afraid of dying has never learned to live...If we are afraid of pain, we can handle it through Christ." I also thought of the words of the Prophet Isaiah, "Surely he took up our infirmities and carried our sorrows...and by his wounds we are healed."[2] I am not alone as I accept my illness as a part of life and live with it. I may not be healed physically, but I can be healed spiritually. This is what keeps the adventure alive.

---

[1] page 126

[2] Isaiah 53:4-5, New International Version

Chapter 6

Adventure Through Acceptance

"How I long for the months gone by
...Oh, for the days when I was in my prime."[1]

Am I to blame for my illness? Am I being punished
for something in my past? Has this illness come
upon me because of my working conditions? Has
my neighborhood made living conditions so
stressful that I have become ill? The above
questions may or may not be a realistic assessment
of the rationalization that goes on in the mind of
one who becomes seriously ill, but they do point up
our thought patterns. Why is this happening to
me? Have I been bad? It's all their fault! Why did
God let this happen to me?

The more important question we should be
asking is, "Now that I have this illness, what am I

---

[1] Job 29:2-4, New International Version

going to do with it?" Shall I be angry about it? Will it help if I blame it on something in the past or blame it on others? Am I just going to cope with it, or should I turn it into an adventure and through it learn more about life? It may be difficult for us to turn our affliction into an adventure; however, we may find it well worth our best effort.

There is a difference between turning an illness into an adventure or just coping with it. I have read numerous books about coping with an illness, or coping with life, and found them helpful and enlightening. According to *The Random House Thesaurus, College Edition*, to cope means: "to contend, spar, wrestle, face, strive, struggle, tussle, hold one's own, manage, hurdle." I am certain that we all do some of these things while trying to improve our condition, and we should. To cope carries the connotation of combat or a struggle to gain the upper hand of the situation. Norman Cousins in his book, *Head First*, gave us some good advice when he said that we should accept the diagnosis but deny and defy the verdict.[2]

On the other hand, an adventure has the element of risk. There are also the elements of the unknown and surprises along the way. There are chances to be taken, and the outcome is uncertain. Experiencing an adventure is something that flows through your very being because you are a part of the happening.

Think back to the time when you were first stricken with your illness. Most likely frustration, anger, resentment, anxiety and fear were present because your way of life had been disrupted. You

---

[2] page 83

were probably thinking, "When will I return to my normal way of life again?" Your response was probably a demonstration of those negative emotions which are counterproductive to recovery. It has been well-established that negative emotions inhibit the healing process.

If the illness is going to be turned into an adventure, there must be an openness and acceptance on the part of the afflicted one. In this unguarded state, the experience itself becomes our teacher, and we can learn the greatest lessons life has to teach us. I am reminded of the statement in Romans 8:13, "I consider that our present sufferings are not worth comparing with the glory that will be revealed in us." Suffering is a part of life, and when it comes my way, even though it is quite foreign to me, I must accept it and learn from it.

I was impressed by reading *The Red Butterfly*, by Linda R. Bell, as she told of her experience with lupus. Here was a young woman whose childhood dreams were unfolding before her in a well-ordered and pre-planned manner. Everything was going her way until she discovered something was drastically wrong with her. Her immediate reaction was to get to a doctor, find a cure, and return to normal life as soon as possible. Isn't that the drive each of us has demonstrated? However, many of us, including Linda Bell, have never returned to what we considered a normal life.

When you realize that you have a chronic illness, you have a choice to make: either to fight and rationalize your condition or to accept it as part of life and learn from it. To accept the situation does not mean that you agree with it or like it. It simply means that you admit it is a part of your life. Now the big question is "How am I going to *live* with it?" Somewhere I have read a statement that goes something like this: *What lies before and behind us is small compared to what lies within us.* All of the emotional reaction to our present life situation lies within us, and this has the potential of being a far greater problem than the illness.

For a few months before I was bedridden with lupus, I thought I was developing a severe case of arthritis. I knew that I was getting progressively worse but didn't realize how bad it was until one day at the auto races at Riverside, California. My younger son, Russell (who had been in Wheeling, West Virginia for six months), and I were track workers at the race. Russ was working pit safety, and I was doing photography. After the race was over, I wanted to climb up onto a three-foot high concrete barrier to get a good picture of the winning driver, but my son had to help me onto the barrier. I shall never forget the stricken look on his face as he said: "Dad, is that you?" My physical condition had deteriorated so much in the six months while he was gone that he hardly recognized me as the man he once knew. Just a few weeks later I was in bed with a low-grade fever.

The early prognosis was rheumatoid arthritis so I pictured myself as becoming progressively bent over with my hands becoming more and more deformed and useless. For a physically strong, athletic person who enjoyed working with his hands, that was a real shocker. I didn't like the thought of it but resolved that if this is what life had in store for me, I would accept it and make the most of the situation. Rheumatoid arthritis was soon ruled out. That was a relief! However, since a diagnosis seemed to evade the doctors despite their best efforts, I reacted with anxiety, anger, and fear during the weeks of tests that followed.

My reaction was probably not much different from yours, "What have I done to deserve this?" Guilt feelings were a powerful influence. Fortunately, I had examined them quite thoroughly before the Visitation Pastor from our church came to the hospital to visit me. He began to raise all kinds of probing questions about my life, thinking that perhaps there was some sin buried deep within that was causing my illness. I looked him straight in the eye and told him, "I have gone over this very thoroughly. I know that my life is not all that it should be. I am like everyone else, there is lots of room for improvement." I further stated, "I am certain that my illness can't be laid to some unforgiven sin." I also told him, "I have read many books and articles on emotionally induced-illness, and I'm quite certain that is not the cause of my present condition." Perhaps this episode contributed to my gaining better understanding of the biblical Book of Job, as Job's three friends tried to find some fault in his life that could be blamed for his physical affliction.

It seems that one of the major problems we face in an illness is that we must fix the blame or cause upon something or someone else. Consequently we get caught in the age old triadic syndrome of "we, they, and me." "We" have done wrong; therefore, I am being punished. This thought is as old as the human race and, by the way, is a major premise in the dialogue of the Book of Job. On the other side is the thought that "they" have done this to me, and again this attitude can be traced back to the beginning of life on planet earth.

Since I did not succumb to the "we" have done wrong and punishment aspect, I could have said, "If `they' (the company) had not insisted that I increase my sales volume each year, I wouldn't have had all the stress which brought on my illness." In either case there is the feeling of betrayal, "I have been shorted in life, either by my past behavior or by what `they' have done to me." This response is precisely because "me" predominates. "Little ol' me, I don't deserve this. Others may suffer, but *why me*?" As I was talking with a man and inquired about his first reaction to his crippling illness of multiple sclerosis, he replied without hesitation, "Why me? Why is this happening to me?"

How do we break this powerful triadic syndrome? Does acceptance mean that our theme song should be "Que sera, sera; whatever will be will be," and passively experience what life has dealt us? No!

Getting well and learning to approach life differently should be the goal of all of us who are afflicted with a serious illness. However, we must realize that we may never be able to live as we did before the illness. This is where the thought of accepting your illness becomes so powerful. We then begin to see life in an entirely new perspective. I would like to illustrate this thought with four living examples; Louie Unser, Donna Nelson, Lillian Haaker and Glenn Main.

Because of my long association with auto racing, I receive a photo pass each year for the Long Beach Grand Prix, giving me access to most of the places I want to go. At many of the races I have seen former race driver Louie Unser on his little electric scooter and his wife, LaVerne, is always with him. Many times I have seen him in the pits talking with his brother Al and other race drivers, but I had never taken the time to talk to him. After my own illness I talked to Louie about his life after the onset of multiple sclerosis (MS). When Louie suspected that something was physically wrong with him, his seven-year journey with twenty different doctors began. He continued racing and, to stay as physically fit as possible, he intensified his physical exercises. Despite all his determined efforts, his physical condition continued to deteriorate. MS affected his vision and crashing into the wall almost became a trademark of his auto racing; he decided that he should stop racing while he was ahead of the game.

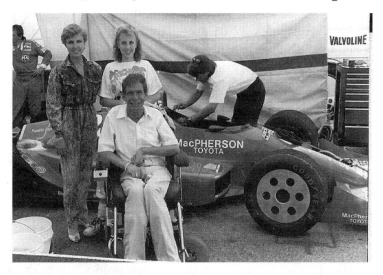

Louie Unser, his wife LaVerne and their daughter Lynn.

As Louie told me about his doctor visits he said, "I had gone to twenty different doctors and each one took a spinal tap. The last one tried several times before he could get it, and I got an infection from it." I said to Louie, "What you are telling me causes me to think that some doctors are no different from some factory workers—they just follow a routine without much thought as to what they are doing."

Some of us will identify with what a doctor finally told Louie. "You seem to have a mental problem, and I am going to place you in an institution for further tests and observations." Some lupus patients have been told, "It's all in your head."

After a few days in the mental institution, Louie told his wife, "I am not crazy. I want you to get me out of here." He told her to get three of his big, husky friends and said, "I don't care if they have to tear the place apart; just get me out of here!"

She came back with his three big friends, who were told they couldn't see Louie. But they found him and, after almost slamming a technician through a wall, they took Louie home.

After recovering from that episode, Louie sought another doctor. He told the doctor about his unhappy experiences with so many doctors and all those spinal taps. The doctor considered all that Louie told him and then said, "Take off your pants. Walk down the hall." The doctor observed the way he walked and asked him many questions. Eventually he told Louie that he might have multiple sclerosis. Just before leaving the doctor's office, Louie asked, "Aren't you going to take a spinal tap?" The doctor smiled and said, "It isn't necessary."

Louie went through the same struggles with anxiety, fear, and anger that we all face. Finally he recognized that he must accept his condition and learn to live his life within it. Louie told me, "Since then, life has taken on a whole new dimension."

Up until this time, building fast race cars and striving to enter the winner's circle was an all-consuming drive. There was no time for others or anything else. Now his thoughts and actions reach out to help others. Eventually, because of Louie's involvement with others who have MS, he was presented the Multiple Sclerosis Father of the Year Award by President Reagan.[3]

I like Louie! In his own unique way he can express himself very simply about his struggles with the thought of accepting his condition. He can talk about how life has changed as a result of accepting his handicap. Later, he will sit there in deep thought and say, "After all these years I still struggle with the thought of accepting my condition." It was not hard for me to understand his struggles. His electric scooter, or a wheel chair, is certainly no substitute for the powerful race cars he has driven. Louie said, "Racing had been my life and I had very little time for anything else. I now see and experience things that were not possible from the cockpit of a race car."

While taking some photographs in the Tech Inspection area at the Long Beach Grand Prix, I noticed a woman doing some of the race car inspection from the seat of an electric scooter. I talked with Donna Nelson and discovered that she

---

[3] Multiple Sclerosis is another auto-immune disease.

had been a healthy, active woman who loved mountain climbing, hiking through the mountains, and also auto racing. Multiple sclerosis changed all of that. She went through the same emotional conflicts we all face. There were feelings of denial; she did not want to surrender her current life-style. She wanted to continue to do the things she had been doing.

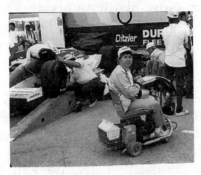

Donna Nelson, on her little scooter, working in Tech Inspection at the Long Beach Grand Prix

Donna is now teaching handicapped children. Some are mentally retarded and others physically handicapped with impaired senses. Donna says that she had known a different life, but these children have never known anything different. She has taken on a new perspective of life as she watches these children manage their lives without really knowing that they are handicapped. She thought, "I am also handicapped, and I must learn to manage my life within my handicapped condition."

I met Lillian Haaker in an art class. I immediately liked her because of her cheerful, outgoing personality. I learned later that she has always been a vivacious and cheerful person even though there had been times when she had wondered if life had been kind to her. Shortly after she and her husband, along with their three daughters, moved from cramped living conditions into a lovely new three-bedroom house, her husband died from a heart attack. Some years later Lillian married a very gregarious man, but that marriage was soon terminated by his untimely death. She found this quite shattering to her sense of security and it also caused considerable emotional upheaval.

Fortunately, she was employed as an executive secretary for a group of engineers in the Advance Design Department at Lockheed Aircraft. To her, working on future development was exciting and helped to ease the pain of the past.

After her girls were married and established their own homes, Lillian remarried. She and her new husband were looking forward to lots of traveling.

About one year after their marriage, she became quite ill. The doctors thought that she had a mild case of multiple sclerosis. It later turned out to be a severe attack of arthritis which left her greatly incapacitated.

When I asked Lillian about her first reaction to her illness, she said, "I was angry, frustrated and embarrassed. I was a bride of only one year—and now this." Because of the loss of her equilibrium, she is in constant need of someone to help her. All of their plans had to be set aside, and she began to ask, "Why me? Why me now?" She said, "I felt singled out from all others because I couldn't keep up with them and was embarrassed to say 'I can't do that anymore.'"

Strong guilt feelings began to emerge as she thought of her anger at the death of her first husband. They had worked so hard, but their plans were interrupted, leaving her with three children to raise. She kept raising the question, "Am I being punished for some of my past?"

Lillian is still quite immobile and has had several surgeries for hip and knee replacements. I asked her how she can remain so cheerful through all of her suffering. She said, "I finally accepted it as a part of my life and thanked the Lord for supporting me in it. Then my attitude began to change." I asked her about the results of accepting her illness. She said, "I have developed a deeper appreciation for my senses, for the things I see, feel, and hear. I see my friends differently than in the past. They are no longer taken for granted—they are deeply appreciated!"

What new dimension of life has come to Lillian as a result of her illness? She says, "I take life one day at a time, and I have lots of time to pray. I depend upon the Holy Spirit to bring to mind others who are in need of help and I pray for them." Lillian says, "One thing I really appreciate as a result of my illness is the deepening of my spiritual life and my relationship to God."

Glenn Main knew there was something seriously wrong with him physically. The doctors eventually told him that he had a tumor on the brain that needed to be removed. I visited Glenn shortly after his surgery and thought that because of his attitude he would soon be home. The doctors and nurses were also pleased with his recovery; then suddenly he had a stroke.

The stroke plunged him into the depths of despair and Glenn began to ask, "Why me?" "Why is this happening to me?" In the depth of that despairing attitude, Glenn said, "Lord, if this is what my life is to be, I will accept it." He now looks back upon the acceptance of his illness as a turning point in his recovery.

Part of Glenn's own personal therapy to recover from his memory loss was to begin memorizing long passages of Scripture. Now that he has recovered and talks about accepting his illness, one would think that he is the first person to discover the value of acceptance. By the tone of his expression, we can almost say that his illness was a great adventure.

This chapter has been written to those who find themselves living with a chronic illness that has come their way and has left them wondering, "Why?" However, there are also illnesses people bring upon themselves due to the way they have been living. Smoking may cause heart problems or lung cancer. Junk food diets contribute to obesity that may also affect the heart. AIDS is a deadly disease that is mainly transmitted by immoral behavior. Many other illnesses could be mentioned. What a psychiatrist friend of mine told me may be apropos. I asked him, "What is the fine line between being mentally healthy or insane?" He replied, "To put it simply in broad terms, if you fill your life with the things that are wrong, you will eventually become my patient. If you fill your life with things that are right, you will never have a reason to see me." Before you draw a wrong conclusion, I should say that he did not intend for his analogy to be all inclusive. I use it to illustrate that some illnesses are brought on by failing to live properly. Regardless of how your illness has come upon you, the remainder of this chapter should be helpful if you are searching for meaning and wholeness in your life.

Whether our illnesses have come upon us as a result of our life-style, immoral conduct, heredity, or apparently from nowhere, there are some lessons about life that we can all learn. We must see the illness as a part of life, whether "I" caused it, "they" caused it, or "it" just happened. You have it and how you respond to it is most important. Good medical insurance or enough money do not always insure good health or recovery from an illness. I have both, yet I am ill.

In other parts of my writings I have addressed the emotional aspect of our illness. I also believe that we must not neglect the spiritual side, regardless of its unpopularity today.

We are living in a day when the almighty dollar seems to rule, and we often completely ignore the spiritual dimension of our lives as we pursue the physical aspects. Could this be the reason for the feeling of emptiness? We begin asking, How can life be meaningful to me in this condition? Has the pursuit of material gain been so important to me? Now that my world seems to be falling apart, do I feel caged with nowhere to go? This is precisely where new life can begin.

We were created in the image of our Creator and, as the writer of Ecclesiastes says, "He [God] has made everything beautiful in its time. He has also set eternity in the hearts of men; yet they can not fathom what God has done from beginning to end."[4] These words come to us from a man of great wisdom and wealth who did not spare anything in the pursuit of pleasure. As he looked for meaning in many aspects of life, he could only say repeatedly, "Meaningless, meaningless, utterly meaningless." His conclusion of the matter was that the real meaning of life is found in a person's right relationship to God.

Our lives are influenced by philosophies[5] that cause us to think that the only thing we can know is what is experienced. They say we can't really know what is right or wrong, good or bad. Truth is only tested by what is practical. We soon take up the motto "If it feels good and makes us happy, then it must be all right." With these philosophies ruling our thoughts, "me" becomes the center of our universe.

If our illness shows us the spiritual side of life, then we are in for a great adventure. We must understand that we cannot satisfy the deeper desires of the heart with only the physical.

Perhaps we can illustrate our dilemma with a passing experience of life. My wife and I live on a mountain pass just east of Bakersfield, California. We had gone to Bakersfield one day when the skies were clear. The valley below us and the surrounding hills were beautiful. The hillsides were bright green and spotted with barren gray oak trees. Some of the fields had a dark border of freshly

---

4   Ecclesiastes 3:11 New International Version.

5   Agnosticism, Empiricism, Existentialism, Hedonism, pragmatism etc.

turned earth. The meadows were highlighted with large areas of bright orange flowers and occasional patches of deep purple lupines.

Amid all that beauty, some of the fields had herds of contented white-faced cows robed in rich coats of red in contrast with the green fields and their beautiful flower patterns. I thought, "Where can one find a more picturesque scene?"

While we were in Bakersfield, the skies turned gray and it began to rain. When we started home, we could see that the mountains were shrouded with dark clouds. As we approached the foothills, one hill stood out spectacularly different from the others. It had deep shades of green with random patches of earth tones. There it stood, contrasted against the stately mountains standing tall with their peaks in the clouds. The mountains looked majestic, robed in deep purple with occasional subtle touches of dark green showing through their purple robes.

The dark skies made the light just right to bring out a beauty that I had never seen before. The fields and wild flowers had deep, bold colors that were spectacular. In another direction, some of the light was filtering through the clouds, painting the hillside in soft pastel colors. Some of the distant peaks were receiving full sunlight, while others were shrouded in the dark grey clouds. What a delightful trip home! This enchanting experience in nature was only possible because of the dark clouds and stormy weather.

At the time I thought, "Here we are, passing through a scene of beauty that I will never see again." I thought of the changing patterns of life and was reminded of the words, "All men are like grass, and all their glory like the flowers of the field. The grass withers and the flowers fall...but the word of our God stands forever."[6] I shall never see that scene again because it is here today and gone tomorrow. However, I know that in the not too distant future I shall stand in the presence of the Creator of all beauty and behold a beauty that can't be described in human language. What a great hope!

Our illnesses may appear as dark grey clouds that we may not like. Others have faced the same thing and have reacted in the same way we have. However, some have learned to look at their condition and accept it. Rays of light have filtered through the dark clouds of illness surrounding them, and they have seen a beauty in life they would not have seen otherwise. What an adventure!

---

[6] Isaiah 40:6-8, New International Version

Chapter 7

Family Adventure

The illness touches the entire family.
Family unity is essential.

Adventure is not only an out-of-doors experience. Adventure may include any new experience or new role in life. I can recall the anticipation that my wife and I had as we waited for our first child. People would often ask, "Is it going to be a boy or a girl?" My fun response was, "Yes! What else would you expect her to have?"

When the moment came to make the trip to the hospital, I realized that all of my anticipation had not prepared me for the event. When I was finally told that we had a girl, I said, "Wow! I'm a father!" My new daughter was the main subject of conversation for the next several days as I proudly told others about my "baby girl." Since then we have welcomed two boys into our family with each bringing a new dimension to the adventure.

The family adventure continued as we watched each of our children adjust to their world and learn from the various aspects of life. Russ, at about age 6, learned that life is not always fair.

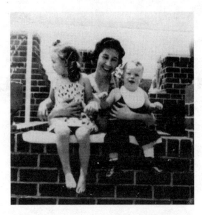

Beth, Audrey, and Samuel

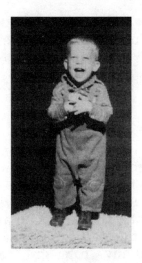

Russell

A baby bird had fallen to the ground. When my young son discovered it, the mother bird took her perch upon an electric wire and scolded and protested his presence. It was not long until our cat put in his appearance, and the mother bird intensified her protest. With angry squawks she dove at the cat, striking him several times. However, the cat was soon on his way carrying the baby bird in his mouth. The mother bird then flew away, and the only one left at the scene protesting was my son. He stood there in pity for the baby bird and angry at the cat as he repeatedly said: "It isn't fair! It isn't fair!"

What happened at that scene is similar to what happens in a family when a major illness strikes. Pity and concern are demonstrated at first, then protests of anger along with the cry, spoken or unspoken, "It isn't fair! It isn't fair!" Regardless of the angry protest, as it was with the mother bird, life goes on.

While the patient is being diagnosed, all the family energy is focused on finding the proper treatment to bring about immediate recovery.

If the person should recover in just a few weeks, the crisis would soon be behind them and life would go on as usual. However, with the chronically ill, everything is extended over time, in many cases for a lifetime. At this stage of the illness, the real family crisis begins with the angry protest, "It isn't fair."

For this portion of the book I have interviewed several families who are living with a chronically ill mate. It is interesting to discover the patterns that emerge from the interviews. A dominant expression by the one who is not ill is anger. The principal reason seems to be that plans have been interrupted, put on hold, or permanently set aside. Projects that had seemed so important will never be completed. Add to this heavy medical expenses and the emotions begin to operate at full strength crying, "It isn't fair! It isn't fair!"

Dr. Parker in his book, *Prayer Can Change Your Life,,* speaks of the four emotions that create a vicious circle within us: fear, anger, guilt and inferiority.[1] He describes fear as the skeleton in the closet. It will set the other emotions into action with each feeding the other, creating a no-win situation. Any one of the above emotions will trigger the others into action.

At the early stages of a serious illness, fear is always present. At a later time, anger will put in its appearance, then guilt feelings will follow, and inferiority is not far behind. It is within this vicious circle that we must fight our individual battles. The family needs to recognize these emotions so that they may keep their thinking and attitudes in proper perspective.

Let me illustrate this with a personal example. I discovered a test that revealed the level of hostility within a person. When I first took the test, my score went completely off the high end of the scale! For three years, I worked on that part of my personality to see if I could become a little more civilized. When I took the test again, I was proud of my improvement. My wife and I were working with a

---

[1] *The Four Demons*, Chapter 5

group of teenagers, and I planned to give them that test one evening. Before they arrived, a full-blown argument developed between my wife, my daughter, and me. I had cooled down (I thought) before the meeting took place. We all took the test and guess what—my score went completely off the high end of the scale! I realized then that when a person is in a state of anger, everything else seems to be out of focus so we cannot come to proper conclusions.

I have been learning that I must deliberately turn from my anger before things can be set right. It helps me when I read from the Scriptures: "In your anger do not sin; when you are on your beds, search your hearts and be silent. *Sela* [Pause and meditate upon this thought.] Offer the right sacrifices and trust in the Lord."[2] Again, "Do not grieve the Holy Spirit of God...get rid of all bitterness, rage and anger... along with every form of malice, be kind and compassionate to one another, forgiving each other, just as in Christ God forgave you."[3] Reading Scriptures, like those quoted, I realized that I must replace anger and rage with forgiveness of others and have a compassionate attitude toward them.

This thought can be illustrated by a retired family who lived across the street from us. The husband was grouchy, angry, and often disagreeable. Possibly he felt that since he had retired his purpose in life had been completed, and now everything was at loose ends. They eventually moved away, and shortly after that we heard that his wife had had a

---

[2] Psalm 4:4-5 New International Version

[3] Ephesians 4:30-32, New International Version

stroke. We visited her in the hospital, and after she was moved to a convalescent home, we made other visits to her. I was pleasantly surprised to see the reaction of her husband. He was cheerful and smiling. As he took his wife for a stroll in her wheel chair, one would think he was courting her for marriage. He would talk to her in tender tones as he patted her on the arm. There appeared to be nothing but love and tenderness between them. I am told that this was almost a daily occurrence for more than two years until she passed away. Anger, malice, and frustration had been replaced by compassion and love. He not only gave me a great lesson in caring for a mate who is chronically ill, but also he was rewarded for his compassion and tenderness demonstrated toward his wife—he was spared the agony of guilt with all of its consequences after her death.

When a person is afflicted with lupus, or any chronic illness, anger is often present in the mate and other family members. It seems that it most often stems from frustration due to a lack of understanding of the illness. Open communication is probably the most direct route to understanding the illness and the emotions that surround it. However, there are times when such communication is painful. This pain may result in denial of the illness and its symptoms.

If there is going to be open communication and respect among family members, each of the members must be given space to handle his own emotions. To be overly protective toward others within the family tends to destroy communication and respect with resultant increased anxiety.

The person with the illness must be careful not to use the occasion as an opportunity to plead for sympathy or to be pampered in any way. It should be a time of seeking to understand how the others feel. When my lupus begins to flare I simply say, "My wolf is snarling at me again." (Lupus is the Latin word for wolf.) That is not a signal for everyone to keep their distance. It is only a nice way of letting them know that I may not be my usual self for a while. After all, they can't tell it by looking at me. Most lupus patients soon learn that they have one thing in common—people often say to them, "You look so good" and think that everything is back to normal. With this assumption, we understand that they will soon demonstrate their impatience toward the ill person who looks good but continues to act sick.

While working on the writing of this chapter I was in my third major lupus flare.[4] As I was leaving church one morning, a man, who did not know that I have lupus, enthusiastically slapped me on the back and said, "You sure do look good! If it's jogging or exercising that makes you look so good, keep it up!" I smiled and thanked him for the compliment, but I was also very much aware of the fact that I barely had the strength to withstand his enthusiastic expression. Each slap on the back almost made my knees buckle.

The family must understand that looks are often deceiving. The person with lupus is not trying to shirk responsibility or find excuses not to cooperate in various things that need to be done. Often the

---

[4] See chapter 11, Emotional Adventure

little things seem almost insurmountable. I was trying to work at my computer one day and just sat there staring at the screen. The task seemed too difficult and confusing. Sometimes the mind just seems to go out of focus. After about half an hour, I gave up. A few days later I accomplished the task in just a few minutes.

Because the mate does not understand what is going on inside a person with lupus, his/her impatience and anger often lead to unbearable arguments, irrational behavior and divorce. Since a larger percentage of women have lupus, we often hear the remark that men are too impatient and intolerant to put up with their wives' long-term illnesses. The husband is accused of soon forgetting the portion of the wedding vows that say to "love and cherish her in sickness and in health as long as you both shall live."

I have news for you! Women have the same problem of which the men are accused. I was in a support group meeting where a man and wife in their mid-thirties were present. The man was quite crippled from arthritis. When he left the room his wife said in an angry tone, "I'm too young for this." It is not uncommon to find anger, hostility, and resentment displayed by the woman because of her husband's major illness. I listened to a Marine tell of his experience in Vietnam that cost him an arm and an eye. After several months of hospitalization overseas, he, along with several other wounded Marines, was placed in an American hospital and their wives were told that they could visit them. The Marine said that after that visit sixty-five percent of the wives walked away, never to see their husbands again. The problem is not one sided, and we all must remember that denial or running away will never solve life's problems.

Illness, pain, suffering, and death are all part of life's cycle. In each phase, it seems we can learn lessons that can change our lives for the better. Isn't that part of the adventure?

Paul and Susan Bond lost their only son as a result of brain cancer, when he was only six and one-half years of age. Paul told me that the traumatic time, even two years later, was still a growing experience. It has caused him and his wife to realize that material gain is no longer the main motivational factor. They are now looking at life entirely differently. He said, "The emphasis is now upon the dearness of life, and there is no way a price tag can be placed upon that." He further stated, "Through this we have learned to communicate with one another more closely than before. We both realized that if we didn't, our marriage would soon break up. We tell each other how we feel and why we feel the way we do. Through this we support one another rather than blame one another." Paul said, "This is a positive way to dispel anger, depression, denial and guilt."

After the death of their son, Paul and Susan decided to adopt a girl, since they could not have any more children of their own. At the time of the adoption they were aware that they might not be able to keep the child. However, for the anticipated joy she would bring into their lives, they were willing to take the risk. They were not only able to keep the girl, but also have adopted another girl. They instinctively knew that the greatest fulfillment of life comes as we invest ourselves in the lives of others.

For those of us who are chronically ill, as we unselfishly do our part to help another, we also contribute to our own well being.

So far we have only addressed the husband and the wife. However, children are also part of the family who must not be overlooked because they have individual needs that must be met also. Fear and guilt take their toll upon them as it does upon the adults.

When a parent becomes seriously ill, the child is likely to have deep feelings of insecurity and fear. The very foundation of the child's life is threatened, and his emotional reaction is just as real as that of the adults. If a child's emotional needs are not met, it may cause him to come to irrational conclusions that may even be carried over into adult life.

It is not unusual for a child to feel guilt because of a parent's illness. Sometimes the child may attempt to take his own life. For this reason some parents have been advised to keep their medicines in a safe place to discourage any attempt by the child to use the medicines for suicide. The children's needs are real and every effort must be made to help them understand.

Many television advertisements lead adults and children alike to believe that there is a pill for every ache and pain. If you use a certain brand of toothpaste, you will never have cavities or bad breath and will always have the best of friends. If you consistently eat the proper cereal for breakfast, you will be strong and athletic with a trim, beautiful body and never a physical care. The advertisements suggest that life can be completely controlled. When a serious and chronic illness strikes, this myth is dispelled.

Another phase of our adventure with a chronic illness is the opportunity to teach our children about illness, medicines, hospitals, doctors, and how to relate to those who are ill or handicapped. The immediate benefits will be a better understanding and sympathy for the one who is ill or handicapped. This may even plant the seeds that will lead some into vocations of social work, health care, medicine, or research in science to meet the health needs of others.

One way to begin the educational process is to change the focus from the illness to the total life situation. Recognize the fact that plans seldom proceed like clockwork to their completion. We all need to understand that adversity and tragedy are often just a step away—yet life goes on. If all of life were sunshine, it would soon become a desert. We need the stormy and adverse times as well, for through them we learn some of the most precious lessons of life.

If it had not been for my own illness, I could not have written even one word of encouragement to others. Throughout my lifetime I have never had patience and empathy for the infirm. One of my most difficult tasks has been to visit someone in a hospital, even a family member. Can you imagine that, even though I am married to a nurse and that I have two sisters who are nurses and a nephew who is a doctor?

Since my illness I have developed an empathy toward those who have an infirmity. Now I find it very rewarding to encourage a person who is ill and to help the family members understand. By talking to the children about a parent's illness and the medications being used, you are also teaching them the various effects of the medicine upon an individual. Children will learn to respect the medicine and seek to understand its effects before they take it for any reason. They also talk to their peers about what they have learned so the educational process continues.

My children were all grown up when I became ill. However, there is one thing I do know and have seen at work in families. When children know that their help is needed, they usually respond willingly. I talked with a friend who has lupus and also two teenage boys. I asked the boys how things had changed at home due to their mother's illness. One of them, whose voice was just beginning to deepen, said in a deep voice: "I wash the dishes and sometimes clean the house." I asked him how he felt about the added responsibility. He replied: "I don't mind so long as it is helping Mom."

I think that is more the norm for the families that are willing to be up front with their children about the illness. Deal with it at each child's level of understanding and don't be apprehensive about enlisting their help.

I am writing from the viewpoint of having the crisis behind you. The patient has been diagnosed and is working with the doctor to get the condition stabilized and the medication regulated. Now it is time to start understanding the total situation.

If the person's illness is lupus, there is apt to be a great deal of misunderstanding by family members because it is very difficult for others to know what is going on within the patient.

Lupus patients may find it disturbing to hear those who are close to them continue to say, "You look so good." It doesn't necessarily come across as positive affirmation. The patient may interpret the statement as saying, "You look so good. Why are you trying to tell me that you are sick? I believe it is all in your mind." As a result of this conflict within the spouse, it may be very difficult to understand why the one with lupus can't carry on as before.

As we look at the over-all picture of life and illness, we not only gain a greater understanding of life but also we bring the family members closer together. Through a better understanding of the illness and its effect upon the entire family, some may embark on a rewarding adventure in life. Why not try it? You have nothing to lose and everything to gain. At this stage it is not appropriate to deny your situation and to run from it. It is not the time to expend your energy fighting against the problem. The time has come to accept it—learn to cooperate with the inevitable and you will be the victor.

Chapter 8

The Support Group

In a support group you will enjoy the benefits
of talk therapy.

I have accepted the fact that I have a chronic illness.
I also realize that many life-style changes must be
made. Where do I go from here? Where will I find
help and guidance as I travel through this maze of
uncertainties? My physical condition, emotions,
understanding my illness, but not knowing what to
expect, taking medicines that I have never heard of,
and all of the other things that enter in seem so
overwhelming. I feel like I am alone on a life raft in
a stormy sea.

What is a support group? Will it be helpful or
detrimental? "I am ill, and if I am around a group
of others who are ill, will that help me? I complain,
and if I must listen to all of the other complaints, is
that going to help me?" You may have many other

questions, and you may not receive satisfying answers to all your questions in a support group. However, there are definite benefits you will receive through your participation. Serendipitous experiences make any adventure come alive with excitement. This may be the very thing needed to stimulate you to better health and understanding.

When I learned that I had lupus I realized that my life was changing. I also knew that, physically, it was not changing for the better. Fortunately, I recalled some of the books that I had read previously and realized that I should read them again. The reading was helpful, for I found direction in living with a chronic condition and also realized that there was hope for the future. This is basically the purpose of a support group, to help you find direction in living with your illness and to discover that there is hope for the future.

When we face a future that is threatening, we do so with fear and trepidation. Fear is one of our emotions that causes us to see things out of perspective. In a support group, we will probably discover that most of our fears are unfounded. Joanna Permut in her book, *Embracing the Wolf*, [1] graphically states why she avoided a support group. She was afraid of what she might see: others worse off than she, or puffed up from the use of steroids, or even resentful because her condition might be better than theirs. One might say that her reasoning was that of fear upon fear. She had heard, through her doctor and others, how support groups had helped others. It was fear that kept her from seeking

---

[1] Page 101

a group. If I had known of a supp
was first diagnosed as a lupus patien.
learned what to expect and how to h
disease from other patients, rather than .
and error.

For the adventurous person, new challenges
new approaches to the "same old thing" always aud
zest to life. Adventure demands that we face what
is new, face our fears, and take our chances. We
must not allow our fears to rob us of the rich
discoveries that are in store for us. Support groups
offer you the experience of seeing yourself through
the eyes of others. This will help to put your fears
and the unpredictable nature of lupus in proper
perspective.

Adults are very reluctant to change their way of
life. We become accustomed to the routine and
seldom leave it unless we are forced to do so. With
most lupus patients, a change of life-style is
mandatory. We do not have to look at a chronic
illness as the end of life; we can view it as a new
beginning. In a support group, you will discover
that many have a personal story about how they
have met the challenge. You will discover that
some have been very creative and found satisfying
new ways of life they never dreamed possible.

Another benefit of the adventure of a support
group is the new friends you will make. Lupus is
no respecter of persons so people from many walks
of life are present and seeking one thing in
common—how do I live with this illness? I can
personally say that my life has been made richer as
a result of the new friends that I have made. I also
trust that I have enriched the lives of others as we

talk about the things we have experienced and what we have done to improve the quality of our lives.

For the person who has just been diagnosed, probably the immediate benefit of a support group is being able to talk about your condition. This is what I call "talk therapy." You need to talk about it, but probably your family and friends don't want to hear any more about how you feel and think that you are just complaining. People in a support group will understand how you feel, know your symptoms, and lend a sympathetic ear.

Help comes when we admit that we hurt and are lonely. Our real need may be not as much physical as emotional; we need someone to walk with us along our lonely path.

One man came to our support group where his hurting was quickly recognized by others. His job was also in jeopardy because of his condition. The group gave him the support he needed, and he left a changed man. Six months later someone reported that he was still a changed man and doing quite well in his employment. Now I call that adventure! I am glad that I was a part of it!

One of the greatest benefits you will receive from a support group is the chance to support another in need. You have gained a degree of success in living with your illness so now you can help someone else. You have also discovered that your change in life-style is not all that bad; in fact, there are facets of it you like. Now you can help others to find their way through their fears and apprehensions.

Talk therapy is beneficial because it allows a person to release pent-up emotions that have been buried because the person may not feel free to release them at home. I was talking with a woman about her feelings and reactions to her chronic condition. Some of the things she told me were with tears in her eyes. She went on and on, just pouring out things that had been buried for a long while. She later apologized for being so emotional and said, "You asked me and I told you. I have been wanting to say this for a long while but didn't have anyone to say it to. My family doesn't want to hear it." This may be the same thing you face. Go to a support group and talk it out!

Another benefit from talk therapy is not only to relieve the pent-up feelings but also to alleviate fears. You will probably discover that others have also faced and have lived through some of the fears that you have about your condition.

A woman was telling me about her daughter's battle with lupus. Her central nervous system was affected and her daughter had been told by her doctor that people with her condition will only live for five years. She was discouraged and wanted to give up. Although the doctor's prediction has been wrong, in a support group she would have been spared the discouragement she suffered and the hopelessness of her condition.

People who have a chronic illness have a lot to overcome. We often need to be spared the well-intended remarks of family and friends when they say, "You must keep a positive attitude." One man said to me, "I am so tired of hearing that remark that I have to use all of my strength to keep from taking a swing at anyone who says that to me."

Family members and friends usually mean well when they make such remarks and don't realize how the patient may react to their "words of solace." Why do they make such remarks? Probably because they don't know what else to say and feel that they must say something. They are trying to be friendly and uplifting and don't know how to go about it.

If the remark is made as a means of giving advice, what comes across is that if you deny your illness you will soon be well once again. Your unspoken or emotional response is, "I am ill and am doing everything possible to recover. Can't you understand that?"

Another statement that is often made without sensitivity is, "It's all part of God's plan." However, this never brings comfort to the person who has been stricken with the chronic disease. Who is that despot that presumes to know God's will for another person? I sometimes find God's will difficult to determine for myself; I am certainly not qualified to determine it for another.

In a support group, you will find freedom to talk about your condition while being spared all of these insensitive remarks. The person who is trying to comfort one who is ill should remember that a listening ear is far more therapeutic than all of the "perceived" good advice one can give. In a support group, there are many listening ears.

In the support group, you have the opportunity to make friends with others whom you may turn to for support and encouragement. When you need help, you can always call them and talk out your problem. I have been encouraged more than once through a phone conversation with another lupus patient. I have also had the privilege of uplifting others in their times of trials. Becoming active in a support group is one of the best therapies you can experience. It is also an avenue of adventure as you work toward gaining control of the illness.

Chapter 9

Who Is In Control?

It's your illness...what are you going to do about it?

There seems to be a two-or three-year period that many lupus patients go through as they adjust to the fact that they have lupus, and life is not going to be what they think of as normal. There is the long period of denial, anger, guilt, inferiority, and far more insidious—self-pity and loneliness. The first group of emotions are part of the emotional battle that we all face. The last two, self-pity and loneliness, are your choice. You may deny this and try to rationalize it to give yourself a little comfort in your misery, but it won't help you.

There are a lot of things that the patient must consider about his/her illness. Probably one of the first things you must face is what your doctor has told you. Your doctor may or may not understand your illness and its effect upon you as I learned in the early stages of my lupus. Earlier, I told you of the medical prescription to treat my illness and the doctor's prediction of returning to work in just a few weeks. Both were unrealistic. Since then, I have often wondered what my illness may have been had I passively followed his instructions. I took the initiative to state my feelings and preferences.[1]

As a result of working with my doctor, he learned more about lupus and how to treat it. I also became a student of lupus and the medicine that is used in its treatment and what to expect from it. It would have been nice to have returned to work as quickly as the doctor thought I could. However, a number of weeks went by before I returned to work and then only part-time for almost a year.

In those few months, I realized that the doctor couldn't cure me. The illness was going to be with me the rest of my life. I could choose to pout about it, or I could choose to take charge of my life and discover a new way of living. The choice was mine. Through my own experience, confirmed through reading and listening to lectures presented by doctors and psychologists, I concluded that I would not feel better until I faced not only my illness but also the emotions that accompany it.

My emotions are where I live. If I want to live a comfortable and respectable life, I must do a little housecleaning. If I allow my emotions to distort the reality of life, no one will care to visit me and I will be a lonely person.

---

[1] Chapter 4, *Me, Chronically Ill?*

How am I going to live with this mess? Settle the question of who is in charge. First of all, your illness belongs to you and you alone, although others around you will have to live with both you and your illness. You are either the person in control, or you will allow your illness to control you. The choice is yours and yours alone. Perhaps the big question you may have at this time is: How do I take control?

You can't control something through ignorance. You must have an understanding of your illness and its effect upon you. It's back to school whether you like it or not. Since many adults resist learning something new unless they are forced into it, it is good therapy to learn about your illness and its effects upon you, and also about the medicine you are taking. Learn how to adjust to others around you. Learn how to listen to your body and make the life adjustments that are necessary so that you may live a life as nearly normal as possible. There is lots of learning to do and the longer you put it off, the longer you will be miserable.

Most of us have a rather narrow exposure to lupus patients and can't speak from a broad view of how others are affected. I know that some have severe physical problems that are caused by the disease. However, many lupus patients I know are carrying on full-time employment. Should the one who is fully employed allow the one who can't work full time tell him/her how to live? Now that may sound a bit harsh; however my reasoning for making the statement is that I have observed this happening. How do we guard against this bad advice?

We must take a broad view of the illness and how others live with it. Lupus is a chameleon that looks and acts differently in different patients. I have become quite weary of hearing some lupus patients giving advice to others who have just been diagnosed, "Don't go out in the sun. Stay away from fluorescent lighting." It is true that many lupus patients are photosensitive; however, I have read that more than half of all lupus patients are not photosensitive. I know one man who just thinks about going out in the sun and becomes ill. On the other hand, I can spend all day working in the yard and the sun doesn't bother me. I also know of many others who are not affected by the sun or fluorescent lighting. Should the one who is photosensitive make another patient a prisoner of his problems? Or should I, not being photo-sensitive, ride roughshod over those who are? No! We should be sensitive to the needs of others and at the same time not take their symptoms and problems upon ourselves. I realize that my condition can change and I could become photosensitive. As a result, I do not throw caution to the wind. I usually wear a hat and never peel off my shirt when working in the hot sun.

At a weekend lupus seminar, I served on a discussion panel with other lupus patients. About two years later, I saw one of the panel members and hardly recognized her. She looked terrible! I inquired about her health, and she told me that her lupus had gone into remission so she had indulged herself in a day of sunbathing at the beach. She has paid a high price for casting caution aside for one day of pleasure.

What works for one may not work for another; therefore, caution should be used. The same thing is true in the matter of the medicine the patient is taking. I have heard pharmacologists say that the medicine that works for me will not work for one-third of others with lupus. What I am saying is that each person must face his/her own set of problems and find their own workable solution. It is helpful when we relate our experiences to others and mutually encourage one another as we seek our individual ways of coming to grips with the illness and learning to live with it.

Many doctors have written books stating that the patients who take charge of their illness recover more rapidly than the passive patients who wait for the doctor to cure them.

This thought is dramatically expressed in the Gospel of John.[2] Jesus came to a gathering of infirm people. He addressed one man who had been an invalid for thirty-eight years asking him, "Do you want to be well?" Off hand, that does not sound like a very good question. Who wouldn't want to be well? Then came the most pathetic reply, "Sir, I have no one to help me...." Later there is an indication that this man was an invalid as a result of his life-style. However, the point is that the man waited for thirty-eight years *for someone to help him* when he should have been helping himself years ago.

Let's take this thought over into everyday life. High blood pressure is sometimes referred to as the "silent killer." It is quite prevalent and doctors say it

---

[2] John 5:2 - 15

is one of the easiest afflictions to control. I have high blood pressure and take medication to help control it. I also like to smell the aroma of fresh brewed coffee and then to savor the taste of it. No doctor has told me not to drink coffee. However, I have learned that coffee constricts the blood vessels and elevates the blood pressure. I have also learned that one of the medicines I am taking for high blood pressure relaxes the walls of the blood vessels and decreases blood pressure. Now, does it make sense for me to continue drinking coffee and defeat what the medicine is intended to do? No! The only sensible thing to do is to stop doing what I like— drinking coffee.

Yes, if I am going to be well, then I must take control of my life so that I move toward wellness. I must take inventory of my total life-attitudes, emotions, spiritual experiences, family, social and physical activities, work, and whatever else I am involved in and properly balance all the elements of life so that I may move toward wellness. If I don't do it, who will? If I wait for someone to tell me, it may be thirty-eight years before anything happens. I would be no different from the man who said, "Sir, I have no one to help me."

It is essential for those of us who are living with a chronic condition to make every effort to control our illness by changing our habits of life so that we will not defeat what doctors are trying to do for us and what medicines are intended to accomplish. The responsibility is ours.

Chapter 10

The Health Care Team

In this part of the adventure, mutual trust must be
earned and communication is essential.

We, as patients, must remember that the doctor
does not have all of the answers to our problems
and is often just as baffled as we are. Our attitude
should be that of working with the doctor rather
than placing unreasonable demands upon
him/her. The scene described below illustrates that
unreasonable demands never help to solve the
issue.

"That's my wife and I want to know what's the
matter with her **now**," were the angry tones that
reverberated in the hospital emergency room as the
woman lay there in excruciating pain. She was
promptly sent to another hospital where she went
through almost two weeks of testing and was
discharged without a positive diagnosis. More than

two years have gone by, and the doctor has said, "I think you may have lupus, but I can't say for certain."

The scene just described is, in some ways, typical of many lupus patients in search of a diagnosis. They want to know *now* what their problem is and become very anxious when the diagnosis evades them. When I was being tested, I felt the stern pressure from the man I worked for, as he tried to persuade me to find another doctor. He, like many others, seemed to have the opinion that if a doctor could not determine the problem in the first or second visit, he was not worthy of the honor of being called "doctor."

From what I have read and also heard others say, it seems that many lupus patients see several doctors before a diagnosis is made. Sometimes their search for a diagnosis covers a few years. Sometimes a doctor will refer the patient to another doctor, often to a specialist. One of the big problems that develops is the lack of communication. Often the patient does not tell the doctor all of the symptoms, and some doctors don't want to listen. Sometimes the patient doesn't think some of the little things are important or may even feel a little embarrassed to mention them. The patient may not want to give the appearance of being a complainer.

When a patient is seeing more than one doctor, one thing that is mandatory is to have one primary health care physician and that he/she have complete medical records from the other doctors. Don't hesitate to ask for them. You have paid for their services, and you are entitled to the records if you request them. You may have to sign a release and have the records mailed directly to the primary doctor's office.

I read the account of one woman who, over the course of a few years, had seen thirty different doctors. There were some doctors who independently came to the same conclusion that she probably had lupus but did not make a positive diagnosis. Finally, she told her story to another doctor who asked her to get the records from all of the doctors she had been to. The latest doctor, after reviewing the records, made other tests that had not been performed previously and finally diagnosed the woman as having lupus.[1]

Often I hear lupus patients say, "I just don't trust any doctor." I ask them, "If you don't trust the doctor, why do you go to him?" So far I have not received a satisfactory answer. Could it be that this lack of trust is the result of poor communication on the part of both the patient and the doctor? Could it also be that the patient doesn't realize that the doctor doesn't have all the answers, and he is expecting too much from the doctor?

The two times I have been hospitalized I have heard some patients give the medical staff verbal lashings because things were not going according to their expectations. I wondered how the staff could tolerate them. We, as patients, must remember that doctors and nurses don't know everything, and they are just as human as the patient. It behooves us to be respectful and courteous to them.

During my stay in the hospital, I was impressed by the teamwork the medical staff displayed. My

---

[1] Beverly Brown, *I Choose to Live*

doctor, in effect, had said, "I have exhausted the tests I am able to perform and don't have a solution. I am releasing my patient to you for further testing and diagnosis."

I was assigned to a health care team and the tests began again. As the team worked with me, they also consulted with other specialists within the hospital. It was very encouraging to see so many working together, each respecting the opinions of the others.

If there is going to be efficient teamwork, courtesy and respect must be demonstrated at every level, and that includes the patient. The patient must recognize that all are working in good faith toward the goal of diagnosing the illness and prescribing the medicine or treatment that is necessary to relieve the pain and inconvenience the patient is suffering and get the patient mobile as soon as possible. To move toward that goal, each must develop an openness and trust, which also fosters good communication.

One thing that will help to develop that openness and trust is remembering that both the doctor and the patient are human. To be human is to be incomplete in knowledge, wisdom and ability in every facet of life. I told you about Louie Unser seeing twenty different doctors, and they appeared to perform like factory workers[2]. That only reveals that doctors, like the rest of us, lack complete knowledge and wisdom. If you find it baffling that your doctor is not meeting your needs, just remember that he/she has a very difficult job to sort through all of the often changing symptoms

---

[2] Chapter 6, *Adventure through Acceptance*

that are involved. This is when it calls for effort on your part so that your thoughts, feelings, and fears may be clearly communicated.

In her book, *Lupus: My Search for a Diagnosis*, Eileen Radziunas reveals the frustration that both she and the doctors faced during her diagnosis. Without question, she endured many tests and even surgeries that were not necessary. One of the surgeries for testing was performed at the request of her primary physician, even though the specialist to whom she had been sent didn't think it was necessary. Finally, she began to state her fears and objections and began questioning whether some tests were necessary.

Much of the frustration that arises in our relationship with the doctor may be due to our lack of understanding and failure to follow the doctor's instructions. For instance, I know of some patients who will refuse to take any corticosteroids because of fear it may give them a puffy appearance. Possibly the question that needs to be settled is, "Do I want to look my best, or do I want to be well?"

On the other hand, I know of doctors who have taken patients off corticosteroids prescribed by another doctor stating, "I don't like the possible side effects of this medicine." When I was faced with this problem, I chose to chance the side effects and to enjoy the effectiveness of the medicine.

In our doctor/patient relationships, we must remember that one doctor will not satisfy everyone who seeks treatment. One of the doctors who I have had was excellent in his understanding of lupus and the treatment of it. I also thought he was excellent in doctor/patient relationships. During a support group meeting, I mentioned his name and immediately one person angrily blurted out, "I would never go to him again!" I simply replied by using the analogy that the medicine that works for one may not work for another and the same thing seems to be true in doctor/patient relationships. We should not condemn a doctor, or all doctors, as a result of our own experience.

We must be careful of stereotyping all doctors, as many patients are prone to do, and speaking disparagingly of them. That doctor who serves you well may not be the best doctor for another patient. I would not want to be responsible for complicating another's illness by my unkind remarks.

While I was discussing doctor/patient relationships with my nephew, who is a doctor, he said that doctors must also trust the patient to tell what is really going on. The doctor must trust the patient to take the medicine as prescribed. When a patient is taking some of the powerful drugs and does not follow instructions, the results could be as disastrous as giving a child a loaded gun. He told me that doctors appreciate it when the patient will take charge of his own health by keeping a record of what is happening within and writing down what he would like to discuss during the next appointment. He also stated that trust is a result of consistent behavior over a period of time. I asked him about patients who are not satisfied with their doctor. He replied that if a patient is not satisfied with the doctor, the patient should tell the doctor rather than a lawyer, or he should find another doctor.

As a pharmacologist addressed our support group, he began with a question: "How many people died of AIDS last year?" There were many guesses and one person almost guessed the number. He then asked: "How many people died last year from not taking their prescription drugs properly?" All of the guesses were way low. We were all amazed to learn that during the past year more people died from not properly taking their prescription drugs than died from AIDS.

He then proceeded to ask individuals: "What drugs are you taking?" "Do you take them with food or without food?" "Why do you take them with food?" "If you forget to take your drugs at the prescribed time, do you take double the amount the next time?" (He advised against that.)

Some were quite uncomfortable during the dialogue with the group. However, he certainly caused everyone to realize the importance of taking his/her medicine as prescribed.

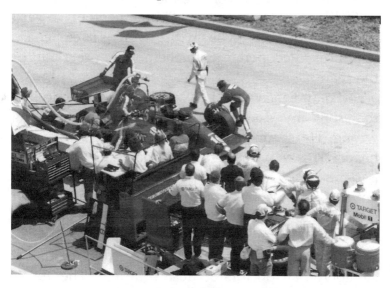

Long Beach Grand Prix—Pit Action

Teamwork is necessary in almost every phase of life. If the family doesn't function as a team, there are problems. When it comes to health care, the basic team is the doctor, the patient, and the pharmacologist. If there is more than one doctor, they should all be considered as part of the team. I can illustrate the importance of harmonious teamwork through my association with auto racing. At one of the California 500 races, I was assigned as tech observer to Mario Andretti's pit, which was between the pits of Al Unser, Sr. and Rick Mears. The tech observers make notations of the times the car enters and leaves the pit and all the events that take place during the pit stop. It is amazing what a team can accomplish in fourteen seconds or less. All run the race, but only one enters the winner's circle. This race was won by less than one second. It was teamwork that won the race.

Health care teams are working together toward the goal of putting you in the winner's circle. Do your best to cooperate with them. You are a part of the team.

You may be saying, "I have been trying to do just that, but my doctor says he can't find anything wrong. He seems to think my problem is in my head." This is a common complaint among lupus patients. Part of the reason for this complaint appears to be, from the patients' point of view, that many doctors are not familiar with lupus, and they don't understand how it affects the individual. Sometimes this is true; however, we should not stereotype all doctors because of a few. The lupus patient must understand that for the doctor, diagnosis can be as evasive as the animal[3] whose name it bears. Lupus is called the great deceiver and the symptoms are often very similar to those of other illnesses.

I was reading a magazine article in which a woman was describing her symptoms and how they physically affected her. I kept saying: "I'll bet she has lupus." Her symptoms were so close to mine that I was identifying with her completely. I felt rebuffed as she concluded the article—she had PMS. I am the wrong gender for that!

In our doctor/patient relationship, we must remember that the patient needs the doctor and the doctor needs the patient. The doctor is just as human as the patient and also has his problems. Sometimes they are just as staggering as the problems the patient is facing; sometimes the doctor's problems have a bearing on how he treats the patient.

Have you ever taken a closer look at the medical community other than your personal visit to the doctor? I was reading a news article about two hospitals that closed their maternity wards. They were fed up with malpractice suits. If a newborn child was abnormal in any way, it was considered the fault of the doctors and the hospitals and they were then a target for a malpractice law suit.

We are all concerned about the skyrocketing costs of medical care and sometimes ask, "Are all of these tests necessary?" Could it be that doctors order a complete battery of tests to protect themselves against malpractice lawsuits?

---

[3] wolf

Dr. C. Everett Koop, past Surgeon General of the United States, commenting on the health care crisis, spoke of the serious deterioration in doctor/patient relationships. He said, "Neither side trusts the other, leading to a situation where the doctor and patient see each other as potential legal adversaries who spark the profession to practice defensive medicine and to pay exorbitant malpractice insurance premiums to protect themselves."[4]

Why am I writing all of this? It is my effort to help us gain an understanding of both sides of the issue so we can work towards better doctor/patient relationships for our mutual interests. I am certain that most of us, from a laymen's view, are not aware of the things the medical profession constantly faces.

My nephew, the doctor, after taking a hard look at what his income must be in order to break even financially, said, "I wish I had been a salesman like my uncle Bob." To meet the expenses of office rent, supplies, staff, and the high cost of malpractice insurance, the amount of necessary income for a doctor in private practice is staggering. And of course, these costs are ultimately passed on to the patient.

I recall reading an article dealing with the malpractice insurance issue. The article stated that very few settlements are awarded to those who sue. However, the insurance companies justify the high cost of premiums on the basis of the large number of malpractice suits, not on how much they pay out

---

[4] *Christianity Today*, September 10, 1990

for malpractice. Greed is never a respecter of persons, nor is it ashamed to be found at any level of life. We all pay the high price for greed.

We must do our part to help reverse the trend that continues to lead to higher health care costs by working toward quality relationships with our health care team. This may also be the difference between a well-managed illness and one that causes needless pain and inconvenience. Be an active participant in the care of your illness. You are the one who will benefit.

Chapter 11

Emotional Adventure

Can the roller coaster emotional experiences be an adventure?

This may sound like a strange chapter title. However, to me, exploring my emotions has always been interesting. While I was in a professional management course, we were asked to take the Johnson Temperament Analysis. The instructor insisted that we work through the process to discover our own personality patterns. There were a few in the class who refused to do it and others who reluctantly went along with it, while some of us eagerly put ourselves into the adventure.

I was required to enlist several others to fill out a questionnaire about me. One went to my wife, another to my daughter, one to a close friend who knew me well, one to a casual acquaintance, and another to a person I worked with. After the questionnaires were completed, it was my responsibility to evaluate them and chart the results in the form of a graph. As I looked at the charted responses, I was pleased. It was as though I were looking in a mirror. It revealed a lot about me that I already knew. However, the greatest value to me was that I saw myself as others see me. The benefit was increased self-esteem which gave me greater confidence in working with other people.

Emotional adventure may sound strange to you; however, we must remember that as we go through life we are on an emotional roller coaster. I shall never forget when I took Sam, my older son, on his first roller coaster ride. The roller coaster train began its steep climb with the rhythmic sound of clog, clog, clog as the gears strained to lift the train to the highest point of the ride. Suddenly, the passengers in the front cars were screaming with delight at the thrill of the steep plunge. At the bottom the wheels groaned as we made a fast climbing turn. I looked at my son and saw his chin pressed against his chest. All of the color had drained from his face. We were violently tossed from side to side as we went through the sharp turns. The wheels continued their loud clackity-clack, clackity-clack as we were ferociously tossed about going over the thrilling ups and downs and through the turns. The passengers screamed with delight all through the ride. I watched my young son's reaction and when it was over I asked, "Were you scared?" Grinning, he looked up and said, "I like being scared." As we explore our emotions, you may at times be afraid of them; however, if you are an adventurous personality, you may also say, "I like being scared."

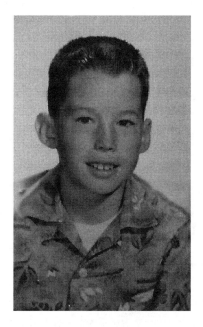

Samuel, 5th Grade

I set aside work on this book for more than a year because I am writing mostly from experience and I needed the time off. Before I started writing again, I read what I had already written because I didn't want this chapter to be repetitious.

As I read through the manuscript, I noticed that I have spoken of my anger and the thought struck me that I may have conveyed the idea that I am a "grumpy old man." That is seldom the case. When I took the Dale Carnegie sales course, two awards were given that most class members wanted: the Sales Talk award and the Human Relations award. Each salesman had a product to sell, and at the end of the course, we took turns selling our product to another class member in front of the rest of the class. The Sales Talk award was given to the one the class selected as having done the best job of selling his or her product. The Human Relations award went to the one selected as having done the most for the class. I missed out on the first one, but was almost unanimously chosen for the Human Relations award. I only say this to correct, if the thought is there, the suspicion that I am a "grumpy old man." I like people, and I like interacting with others.

In various settings, such as church groups, business encounters, classroom occasions, or just casual encounters, I have often had people tell me, "You set me at ease in your presence." One time when I was the moderator for a lupus seminar, I was amused at the comment of one woman. She said, "You must be fun to live with." I was talking about this with my wife and said that I may have communicated the thought that I am a "grumpy old man," and she said, "Well, I still like you." Now that is something! After almost a half century of being married to the same woman, she still likes me! Perhaps all of this is overly emphasized, but I didn't want you to have a wrong impression of me and discount my ideas because of what I have written about anger. I am loved by God, I like myself, and therefore, I can love you also. I feel that I have something to offer.

Psychologists have used different ways to describe the human personality. Karen Horney in her book, *Our Inner Conflicts*, has said there are basically three types of people: those who move towards people, those who move away from people, and those who move against people. The ones who move toward people can best be described as needing to be loved. They will do anything to win your love and approval. Those moving away from people are the ones who tend to be loners and even the suggestion of a helpful book would be regarded as an intrusion into their private lives. Those who are moving against people are the aggressive ones where the underlying mood is that of anger. They are the movers in life. They get things done regardless of what it takes.

Another analysis of the personality is based on the four temperaments and the various combinations of them. They are: sanguine, choleric, phlegmatic and melancholy. The sanguine and choleric are outgoing personality types, while the phlegmatic and melancholy are introverted. For a brief description of the sanguine, one could say that this person is the "life of the party." When Miss Sanguine arrives, everything becomes lively, upbeat, and jovial. When Mr. Choleric is present, things begin to happen. He knows where he is going so don't bother him with details. He is likely to walk all over you in the process, but he will get the job done. Mrs. Phlegmatic comes along and wonders, "Why all of the fuss? There's lots of time to do what needs to be done. Why are you in such a hurry?" She likes to take time to smell the flowers and enjoy the scenery along the way. To her, what difference does it make whether she arrives at her destination today or next week? Ms. Melancholy arrives on the scene and if all the plans have not been made and the details nailed down, she is upset and very insecure. She wants to know all of the details. When Mr. Choleric and Ms. Melancholy are in close working relationship, a full-blown confrontation often develops because they are working against one another.

All of these temperaments are good and needed for the benefit of society. However, the ones who cause the most problems for themselves are the choleric and the melancholy. The one who is most likely to have a heart attack or a chronic illness is the choleric. The choleric personality tends to be driven; he does not take sufficient time for rest and relaxation. I am basically a combination of choleric and sanguine with the choleric predominating. My wife is basically melancholy and phlegmatic. These opposites are the basis of most of our conflicts. W e each need the other to round out what is lacking in our individual personalities. When this is understood, we realize that the differences can be mutually beneficial.

There is also another description psychologists use to describe personality traits: **type A** and **type B** personalities. Using this description, the **type A** would be basically choleric and the **type B** personality basically phlegmatic. Another way to describe the **type A** personality is that this person is always in a hurry and overloaded. If the **type A** person is carrying in the groceries, he will try to take more bags than he can carry and usually drops something along the way. The **type B** person will carry them in one bag at a time regardless of how long it will take.

You have probably heard of the analogy of the tortoise and the hare. Or, to put it another way, the race horse and the turtle. We basically need to determine, "Am I a race horse or a turtle?" If you are the race horse, **type A** personality, you are a prospect for the diseases that may be triggered from what one psychologist has termed "hurry sickness."[1]

You may be wondering how I view myself in the light of the above descriptions. I may be described as one who is moving toward people until crossed. Then the other side of me takes over, and I am moving against them. The underlying mode of moving against people is that of anger. I am a mixture of sanguine and choleric. In group settings, I am often a sanguine personality. However, when I am task-oriented, I am definitely choleric. This does not mean that I have a multiple personality. Both phases are integrated into one personality. This means that I know who I am and how I work and interact with others and the effects that I have upon them. I also recognize that my personality type and life-style have made me a good candidate for an illness such as lupus.

You may be asking; "Why should I learn about my emotions? What do they have to do with my illness and my getting better?" You need to learn about your emotions because of the effect they have on the immune system. Therefore, it is essential for better health to understand and control your emotions. A chronic illness is said to have its emotional stages: denial, anger, depression, bargaining, and reconciliation. If you are going to

---

[1] Archibald Hart, *Adrenalin & Stress*

gain control over your emotions, it is important that you recognize the emotional stage you are in.

When I was in sales work, I was aware of the value of what I learned from the Dale Carnegie sales course. We were taught that every sale will go through five definite stages, and to me it was important to know what stage the sale was in. Why should I try to close the sale if I hadn't convinced the buyer that my product was needed and beneficial to him? I believe the same thing is true for the person with a chronic illness. Know the emotional stages you pass through, and you will be able to respond appropriately and be more at ease with yourself and others around you.

Denial is usually the first reaction. "No, this can't be happening to me." As I read the book, *Embracing the Wolf,* by Joana Permut, it seemed that she was in the stage of denial for about two years. She didn't like the sound of the word "lupus," and she didn't want anything to do with support groups. She denied almost everything except the fact that she didn't feel good and could not function as she had previously. Denial is basically an attempt to alleviate an internal conflict, not wanting to accept the awareness of how we feel.

Teresa Hoffman was ill and discouraged so I gave her the chapters I had already written for this book, asked her to read it and let me know if it helped to encourage her. When she returned it to me, there were notes all over it. Many of her suggestions have been included because I valued her insight. After I had written this chapter, I gave it to her to read. When I received it back, I discovered a note about her denial and anger that I thought should be included. She said, "When I was told I had Chronic Fatigue Immune Deficiency, I was angry with the doctor. I felt he didn't know what was wrong so he just stuck me under this heading. That was total denial."

Through working with lupus groups, I have seen others who want to act as though they don't have lupus. Some have even requested they be dropped from our mailing list for fear it might get into some of their records related to employment and/or insurance. They feared they might be suspected of having lupus if they had received the newsletter. Denial will push the patient to irrational decisions and behavior.

When a person is denying the disease, they often don't want to take their medicines and firmly state, "I don't want that medicine in my body." But, if untreated, the illness will only get progressively worse and eventually cause all kinds of complications. In some cases, serious surgery may be required to correct their state of health. Really, is denial worth it?

Anger usually accompanies denial and is also an expression of our anxiety. For the chronically ill, the root of it is probably a feeling of inadequacy. It is not uncommon to become angry at God, with the doctor, and toward the employer. Anger may also run rampant within the family. It just seems to spill over into every facet of life. One helpful thought: you are not alone when it comes to the display of these emotions. Most of these negative emotions are produced from a feeling of inadequacy to face the conflicts that are raging within us. Anyone with a chronic illness must work his or her way through the emotional spectrum.

As I look at the emotions we experience, I believe that anger is the most devastating. I am embarrassed as I look back upon the times I irrationally displayed anger toward others. It was anger, though at the time it seemed justified, that caused my most serious lupus flare.

Our County Supervisor used to have community breakfast meetings once a month. At one meeting, he was telling about the ninety-three million dollars the county had to return to the taxpayers. Some of it was allocated to special districts such as parks and recreation district, hospital district, community services district (CSD), etc. It was the district's responsibility to request funds for specific projects. He asked one community services district manager to tell about the $250,000 his district received. Afterward I asked, "What did the Golden Hills CSD receive?" He asked, "What did you ask for?" Immediately I knew the answer. I knew that our manager didn't ask for anything. I was a member of the CSD board of directors—and I was angry! The board hadn't been informed of the opportunity. That afternoon I had a doctor's appointment and when he saw my blood pressure reading he said, "You are either very angry about something, or your blood pressure is getting out of control." Since he lived in our community, I told him about the Supervisor's meeting, and before I left his office, he was also angry.

At the next board meeting, it was discovered that our manager had received the letter stating that grants were available to the district upon request. He didn't know what to do about it so didn't do anything. I wanted action to replace him; however, the other board members chose to excuse the matter and swept it under the rug. My reaction to the whole thing was an angry campaign against the CSD that extended over a period of time. There were beneficial changes made within our community services district as a result of what happened. However, I paid for my rampage of anger by spending another three months in bed with my second lupus flare. Was it worth it? No!

During that three months of down time, I learned some good lessons, but it is not easy to write about them.

I had taught the Book of Revelation to a home Bible class for men and was preparing studies in the Book of Isaiah.

I had been in the lupus flare for almost a month when one morning I was reading Isaiah 14. My mind seemed foggy, and I was having a tough time letting things register as they should when I read, "The grave below you is all astir to meet you at your coming; it rouses the spirits of the departed to greet you...They will all respond, they will say to you, `you have also become as weak as we are; you have become like us'".[2] At that moment, the hospital tape that I had listened to about five years previously began to play in my mind. "Systemic Lupus Erythematosus is a chronic illness and there is no known cure. Life expectancy is about five years...." You can understand why I was shaken at that time. I discontinued reading from Isaiah for the time being and asked the Lord to direct my thought to something that would be helpful to me.

---

[2] Isaiah 14:9-10, New International Version

The Book of James is a book of action I have always enjoyed reading because it gets to the heart of the matter quickly. Since it came to mind, I felt that I should read it once again. When I read, "Who is wise and understanding among you? Let him show it by his good life, by deeds done in humility that comes from wisdom. But if you harbor bitter envy and selfish ambition in your hearts, do not boast about it or deny the truth. Such `wisdom' does not come down from heaven but is earthly, unspiritual, of the devil. For where you have envy and selfish ambition, there you find disorder and every evil practice. But the wisdom that comes down from heaven is first of all pure; then peace-loving, considerate, submissive, full of mercy and good fruit, impartial and sincere. Peacemakers who sow in peace raise a harvest of righteousness."[3]

The moment I read those Scriptures I knew that it was touching on the heart of my problem. I was not living by the "wisdom of God" and as a result there was disorder and evil practice. I did a lot of soul searching and also began to get better. I was pleased with the recovery I was making and then my lupus flared up again. I said, "All right Lord, what do you want to teach me now?" The reply, "You have not yet learned what I am trying to teach you about anger. Stay down a little while longer."

The Bible says a lot about anger and its control, including the necessity to turn from it. After a few more weeks of being on the bottom physically, I was gaining new ground spiritually. The words of a quote came to mind, "There were two men in a

---

[3] James 3:13 - 18, New International Version

prison cell—they looked out through the bars; one saw the mud and the other saw the stars." This was true of my experience. I looked out through the emotional bars of my life, and I saw the wisdom of God among the stars.

Henry Gariepy in his book, *Portraits of Perseverance* , in a chapter entitled "A Conscience Without Reproach," says that our conscience is always on watch, always ready to warn us of danger, and he describes conscience as "condensed character." He says, "Self interest asks, `Is it gratifying?' Expediency asks, `Is it advantageous?' Caution asks, `Is it safe?' But conscience asks, `Is it right?'" He went on to say, "A bad conscience embitters the sweetest comforts; a good one sweetens the bitterest crosses."[4]

What makes the difference between a bad conscience and a good conscience? According to James, if our wisdom is according to this world, ruled by envy and selfish ambition, we can expect negative results. On the other hand, if we display the "wisdom from above," there will be purity of life, we will be peace-loving, considerate, submissive, full of mercy and good fruit, impartial and sincere. Wow! I had a problem! I am truly thankful for the grace of God that works within to remold me into a new person.

There have been times of irrational anger since then, and my conscience has asked, "Do you want to spend another three months in bed?" I am thankful for those warnings and also for the ability to respond in an appropriate manner.

---

[4] Page 143, 144

Depression is another severe emotional stage that we all pass through. Some have referred to depression as being our emotional waste basket. The result is often deep discouragement. It is an unpleasant reaction that gives us a signal that something is seriously wrong. Its causes may be physiological, psychological, or a combination of both. It may arise from conflicts within due to the unrealistic demands we make upon ourselves that result in a sense of failure and a deep feeling of despair.

One of the great dangers that accompanies depression is suicidal tendencies. Recently, I heard a young woman say that she has been suffering a lot from depression. She further stated that although she had never been suicide-prone, she now has had many thoughts of suicide. She is seeing a doctor for treatment of depression. I could identify with her because I had also gone through that stage and also had thoughts of suicide. At that moment if there had been an appropriate way to bring it about, I would have been very tempted to end my life.

I know that for severe cases of depression, especially if there are suicidal tendencies, the patient should seek professional help. There are medications that can be prescribed to help the patient work through his/her depression. However, I believe in the final analysis the person must come to grips with his/her depression and adequately deal with the matter.

With the chronically ill, depression may be the result of your body telling you that something is seriously wrong, and you are feeling helpless to do anything about it. Accompanying the feeling of helplessness is the lack of self-worth and hopelessness. You feel trapped and there seems to be no way out.

Dr. Rolland Parker in his book, *Emotional Common Sense,* said that writing the chapter on depression was harder than any other chapter of the book because there are so many causes of depression. He also gives fifteen suggestions for handling it.[5] All but one call for action because activity is the opposite of depression. Some of his suggestions are: avoid loneliness; get your mind off yourself; stop negative thinking; redevelop hope in other areas.

The suggestion I like best is "enjoy your depression." How does that grab you? He says, "I try to experience it as deeply as possible...I look at depression as a form of rest. It's taxing to take action all the time." The thought of enjoying depression appeals to me because it fits my personality. It opens the door for appropriate change since change must come from within.

No one is immune from inner conflicts. When they are not resolved, the result is depression. When the causes are identified and resolved, renewal and transformation take place. Depression is difficult to deal with. I strongly suggest that you find a copy of Dr. Parker's book and read the chapter "Understanding and Overcoming Depression."

Bargaining is an emotional stage that is mostly an exercise in futility. I like to think of this stage as "foxhole religion." During World War II, it was not uncommon to hear of people who made promises

---

[5] *Emotional Common Sense,* page 120

to God during the fierceness of battle, who when
they went for rest and recreation lived as though
God did not exist. Bargaining is a useless exercise
that leaves a person with only guilt feelings. I am
fortunate that in my illness I never bargained,
"God, if You will only let me get well, I will be this
or do that." If I had bargained, I probably would not
have fulfilled my end of it and then would have
suffered guilt and inferior feelings for having
failed.

Reconciliation is a wonderful stage of the illness.
You have made peace with your illness. You still
have it, but you are no longer fighting it. You have
decided that it is part of your life. Now you can live
once again. Beverly Brown in her book, *I Choose to
Live,* tells of the many doctors she saw as she
struggled for a diagnosis, while now she is living
with her illness. The title of the book and her
concluding words speak of her resolution—"I
Choose to Live."

Why have I spent so much time on the
emotions? Because I think my emotions have
played an important part in my lupus flares. Our
emotions, especially negative emotions, have a
negative impact upon the immune system. Since
lupus is considered an auto-immune disease, your
immune system needs all the help it can get. One
way that you can help is to gain control of your
emotions. You may ask, "How do I do that?" There
is no substitute for reading about emotional
behavior to gain an understanding of your inner
responses. Take an inventory of your feelings
because the experiences of life ultimately are
perceived in the realm of feelings. They are the
scales upon which we measure and value our lives.

Recently, when I went to my doctor for a check up, she looked at my chart and said, "You haven't had any medication for lupus for more than two years. How do you account for that?" I told her that I had been in remission for more than two years and believe it was because I had followed a very definite formula. She asked me to tell her about it. I told her that I believe that if a person with a chronic illness will get the proper medical care; get sufficient rest; eat a well-balanced diet; gain control of the emotions, including stress; and allow space and time, I believe the illness will go into remission. She agreed with my observation. Since then I have read almost the identical thing in a book written by a medical doctor and another written by an osteopath.[6] I believe it is a good recipe for anyone with a chronic illness and also believe that the majority of lupus patients will experience improvement, perhaps even remission, for long periods of time, if not permanently.

I am aware that with some chronic illnesses the patient's condition will get progressively worse. You should not feel guilty or inferior if your condition does not improve. But from all that I have read about illnesses and chronic conditions, the *majority* of patients can expect significant improvement, with long periods of remission, even the possibility of permanent remission. Doctors have stated that the body has an incredible capacity eventually to heal itself. If the body is going to heal itself, your cooperation is necessary.

---

[6] Bernie Siegle, *Peace, Love and Healing*

Robert S. Ivker, *Sinus Survival*

Adequate rest and emotional relaxation must have a high daily priority. You will probably not observe major changes next week. However, you may look back five years from now and say, "Wow! There has been a significant change in my condition."

I will enumerate the five ingredients once more to help you remember them:

1. Get proper medical care. The chemical imbalance of your system needs help.
2. Get sufficient rest which is necessary for physical and emotional restoration.
3. Eat a well-balanced diet to help you gain strength and aid the healing process.
4. Gain control of your emotions and stress. Negative emotions block the healing process and stress will rob you of the rest you need.
5. Allow time (years?) for the illness to subside. You were probably a long while getting to your present state of health, and it will also take a long while to recover.

There is one other aspect of the emotions that should be addressed. Doctor Archibald Hart in his book, *Adrenaline & Stress,* speaks about adrenaline addiction. Some type A persons become so enthusiastic about life that they are often on an emotional high. They become addicted to their own adrenaline and enjoy it, just as the drug addict is addicted to the high from the drugs he takes. It is important for us to understand that overproduction of adrenaline will produce extreme stress in the body.

One time I was on an adrenaline high for a number of weeks because I was so enthused about a project I wanted to see happen. It was a project that involved both business and a church. The church was seeking land for a building site, and I discovered some acreage that seemed perfect. Some of the acreage was zoned commercial and the church could have sold it for businesses. The church could have eventually come out of the project with its portion debt-free. The deal was attractive because it was almost a distress sale. The owner had to sell or within a few months he faced a tax lien sale or foreclosure. Without advertising, I had two business people approach me about buying portions of the commercial area. However, the project seemed too big to the church. Since none of them had done anything of the sort before, fear and uncertainty ruled the hearts and minds of those who had to make the decision. It didn't go through because it would have required the church to put up a large sum of money to get things moving, and they felt the risk was too great. As a result of my extended adrenaline high and frustration, I was in bed once more with a third major lupus flare.

The important thing for us to remember is that the body can't tell the difference between adrenaline high (stress) and the negative stressors we experience. We must be on guard at both ends of the spectrum.

Yes, exploring my emotions has been and continues to be an adventure. As I look at my life in all of its complexity, physical, emotional, and spiritual, I must agree with the words of the psalmist, "I praise you [God] because I am fearfully and wonderfully made; your works are wonderful, I know that full well."[7] Twelve years ago I was told that I had a five-year life expectancy. I wouldn't trade my past twelve years for all of my previous sixty-two years. It has been a great adventure!

---

[7] Psalm 139:14, New International Version

Chapter 12

Adventure Through Humor

Why take life so seriously, you can't get out of it
alive anyway.

After a long discussion about our emotional life,
perhaps it's time for something on the lighter side.
A little humor always helps to lighten the load and
ease the tensions.

I can recall when, in the work place, small posters
with catchy sayings were popular. I remember one
that read: "Why take life so seriously, you can't get
out of it alive anyway." Even in the depths of our
illness, we can still find humor that will help to
ease the emotional conflicts and aid the healing
process.

Humor covers a broad spectrum: jokes, wise
cracks, jesting, the ridiculous, ludicrous, slapstick,

low humor (on the dirty side), wittiness, satire, or just the mood of the person.

I have found that the use of humor is a pleasant way to soothe pent-up feelings, gain new friends, approach a difficult task, break down barriers in relationships, promote business in difficult times, and also to meet the challenge of a devastating illness.

When I went into the hospital for surgery I thought: "I don't like the idea of being hospitalized. What can I do to lighten my time there?"

I took along a few gimmicks hoping to provoke a laugh out of some. The only problem was that I just didn't feel like using any of them until one evening when a patient was giving the nurse a bad time. There were four of us in the same room and everyone was asking the guy to "cool it!"

Finally, as the distraught nurse was leaving the room, I called her back. I had taken a bloody and gruesome looking rubber sore thumb to the hospital with me. (I often used it when I gave talks for various industries to stress the importance of hand safety.) I had slipped the rubber thumb onto mine and was lying there holding my hand as though I were in pain and said, "With all of the commotion going on, I raised my bed to see what was happening and got my thumb caught in the mechanism."

She looked at the thumb and bolted for the door saying: "I'll get a doctor." Just as she went out the door she stopped, pointed a finger at my thumb, and said, "That's not real!" I replied, "I was just trying to put a little humor into a bad scene." Everyone, including the nurse, was laughing, and the mood of the room changed from that of tension to a relaxed atmosphere. The next morning the head nurse came in and asked, "How is your sore thumb this morning?" It was interesting that the story had made the rounds and amused those who weren't even present.

The humor that I find satisfying and beneficial is one that flows naturally. I guess one can say that it is the mood of the person; the ability to see the sometimes incongruity of life.

Humor is good medicine and is needed. Someone has said that a good belly laugh is internal jogging. A person always feels good after a good belly laugh, even if that person is the butt of the humor.

I recall a party that our church group in Ramona had when I had been there for a short time. One man who was new to the group wanted to involve us in a game. He passed out a slip of paper to each person saying: "There is something written on both sides; don't look at the other side until I tell you".

The first side was to be a warm-up time, and each of us did our assignment separately: crow like a rooster, hop like a kangaroo, moo like a cow, etc. Then he asked everyone to look at the other side of the paper and when he gave the word, everyone was to do what it said all at once. On every slip of paper, with the exception of one, it said, be quiet. He had deliberately given me one that said, bray like a donkey.

I got myself ready to outdo everyone. I slouched down in the seat with my legs stretched out and my head laid back. He gave the signal for us to perform, and I let it roll with all that I had. As I brayed away, I realized that all the others were quiet, but I couldn't stop braying. I finally started laughing and laughed until my sides ached. Later the man said he had just wanted to find out what kind of person I was. That was the beginning of a very good friendship.

When I was an industrial salesman with Snap-On Tools, we had annual sales conventions. Different salesmen were often asked to give a presentation on various aspects of our work. One year I was asked to do something on closing the sale. It was left to my discretion and creativity as to what I would do.

The next year, just two weeks before the sales convention, my branch manager said: "You are to present something on closing the sale." I told him, "No, I did that last year." He said: "Do it again". I had a hard time getting enthused about it because I didn't think that was a very important subject for industrial salesmen. Our job was to sell, and it was the purchasing agent who closed the sale. If we didn't do a good job of selling, he would not close it in our favor.

Since Western Division management had been bombarding us with short articles about closing the sale, I decided that I would like to get their minds off that subject, so this time I used a very simple approach to using the hour that was assigned to me.

As I addressed the group I said, "Last year I was assigned the topic of closing the sale and I have the same subject again this year. I don't know whether last year's performance was so great that you want a repeat performance, or that I bungled it so badly that I can be compared to the hit man who got a contract to blow up a car—he burned his lips on the tail pipe."

I thought the group would never stop laughing. Fifteen minutes of my hour passed quickly, and everyone was in a jovial mood. By the use of humor, they were well prepared for what would happen in the next forty-five minutes. I laid my job on the line as I said, "Each year someone is asked to make a presentation on closing the sale. This year we were bombarded with short articles about closing the sale. As industrial salesmen, I am wondering how many sales you actually close."

There was silence for about ten minutes, and I was prepared to stand there for the whole time allotted to me and wait. Finally, the top salesman from the Seattle area spoke up and stated that he probably did not close more than five percent of his sales. Then others spoke up and told how few sales they actually closed.

As my time was up, I summed it up by saying: "What you have expressed is also my experience. I wonder why this is perceived to be such an important aspect of our work that we must cover it each year." That was the last time the subject was addressed. If I hadn't approached it with humor, it probably would have been a disaster.

Norman Cousin's book, *The Anatomy of an Illness*, was popular about the time I was diagnosed, and he stressed the importance of laughter. Through his own self-directed experiment he proved to the doctors that laughter could reduce the sed-rate and improve the physical conditions. While Beth was looking for ways to make me laugh again, she discovered a TV program entitled "Bloopers" and thought it would be good for me. Well, I dragged my bones out of bed to watch the program. It was mostly slapstick type humor that has seldom appealed to me. I was back in bed long before the program was over.

After being diagnosed with lupus, it seemed that many people wanted to keep their distance for fear it was contagious. Here again I used humor to break down the barriers. When I would say that I had lupus I noticed that most people would say: "Uh hu," then after a while trying to puzzle it out, they would say, "What's that?" I had learned about how long it took before they would say, "What's that?" and could say it in unison with them. That always got them to laughing and eased the reticent feelings that were there.

At that time lupus was spoken of as a connective tissue disease, so I told them: "It is an inflammation of the connective tissue of the body. The connective tissue is the cellular glue that holds us together." They would ask, "How is it treated?" I would reply, "Since I am coming unglued at the cells, I am taking a tablespoon of Elmer's Glue three times a day so that I can get glued back together." That usually got a good laugh and also served to break down the wall of suspicion that I might pass something on to them.

Humor is a creative and a pleasant way of dealing with an illness. I know that there are days when a lupus patient can hardly think, let alone see anything humorous in life. It's the better days when humor can be applied, and it helps break the tension that we face while seeking to overcome our illness.

We should never underestimate the power and benefits of humor as part of the great adventure of life. Some will remember when Burma Shave had its humorous signs along the well-traveled highways which broke up the sometimes monotony of driving.

The background of Burma-Shave is interesting. Mr. Odell, founder of the Burma-Vita corporation, was an attorney. However, he needed more income than his law practice brought in, so he started manufacturing liniment in his law office. He learned his recipe from an old sea captain. The vital oils for it came from the Malay peninsula and Burma, and "Vita" from the Latin word for life and vigor—the whole name meaning "Life from Burma."

To advertise his product, he thought up the idea of using humorous jingles along the roadside. The verse had to be read over a distance, and each sign that made up the jingle had just a few words on it. Some of them might be good for our fast pace today. One series of signs read:

Past/ Schoolhouses/

Take It Slow/

Let The Little/

Shavers Grow/

Burma-Shave.

The company met the challenge of the electric razor with the same type of humor.

A Silky Cheek/

Shaved Smooth/

And Clean/

Is Not Obtained/

With A Mowing Machine/
Burma-Shave.

Sometimes the verse appealed to romance.

She Kissed/
The Hairbrush/
By Mistake/
She Thought It Was/
Her Husband Jake/
Burma-Shave.

When there was a crusade against drunk driving, a series of signs appeared:

Drinking Drivers/
Nothing Worse/
They Put The Quart/
Before The Hearse/
Burma-Shave.

As business increased and he needed a wider variety of jingles, he started a nation wide contest to create new ideas. The response was overwhelming, and his business continued to prosper even during the great depression. He employed the pleasant use of humor to get nationwide involvement to help him promote the prosperity of his business, while during that same period many other businesses failed.

I have discovered that if I depend upon jokes for humor I usually end up on the short end of things. Once I was on staff at a youth camp at Prescott, Arizona. All week long I had other staff members laughing. The director of the camp asked me if I would tell some jokes at the special meeting on the last night in camp, and I agreed.

During the dinner hour I was introduced as the "funniest man in camp" and that I would tell a few jokes. My big weakness was that I could never prepare for this type of performance. It just had to flow spontaneously.

I got up before the kids and couldn't think of a single joke. I thought if I made one up it would start other jokes flowing. So I made up one about my cat; it was partly true but mostly fiction. The kids got so involved with the cat that when I turned it into a joke they were feeling so sorry for the cat that they couldn't see the humor. Well, so much for the "funniest man in camp"!

I have used these illustrations, not to teach you how to create humor, but to emphasize that humor can be found in unexpected places, and we can use it to benefit ourselves and others. For me, humor is a vital part of my adventure, whether it be with friends, in business, or living with a chronic illness.

Chapter 13

The Work Place

It is God's gift that all should eat and drink and take
pleasure in all their toil.[1]

A major issue one with a chronic condition must
face is that of employment. Shortly before I
returned to work, my field manager wanted to talk
with me so I invited him to my home for lunch.
We talked about many things, and then he raised
the issue of retirement. I perceived it as a threat and
quickly replied that when I felt it was time to retire
that I would be the first to mention it. I liked my
work, the company I was working for, my fellow
employees, and my customers. I was not ready to
leave all of that behind.

As I returned to work, there were problems in
adjusting to my limitations. I would begin the day

---

[1] Ecclesiastes 3:13. New Revised Standard Version

with enthusiasm, but by noon I could hardly move. I had to learn what I could and could not do and pace myself to just live one day at a time. It was not only a learning experience for me, but also for the branch manager.

Shortly after I returned to work, several school districts were having an industrial teachers convention and their suppliers were asked to set up display booths of their products. I always enjoyed these times because it was a good opportunity for showmanship in sales, and I looked upon that as one of my specialties. It was also an appropriate place to interact with our customers. To me, good customer relationships were the foundation of my business. The show also provided a time to see our competitors and learn more about their ways of doing business.

I was asked to organize and set up our display booth and schedule the times for the other salesmen to work at the booth. The convention was only three days, but they were long days. Because of my enthusiasm for that kind of duty, I had the strength to do it. However, after it was over, I spent the next three days in bed recuperating.

When I talked it over with our branch manager, he was very understanding and said, "I will never lay something like that on you again." He also agreed with me that if I needed shorter days for a while that it would be all right. I guess I was fortunate to be associated with Snap-On Tools where employees were valued as a great asset to the company, and managers were willing to work with employees to meet their needs.

Since then I have read about other lupus patients and how their employers were patient with them until they were diagnosed. Then they started procedures to terminate their employment. Often the employer would not accept the patient's diagnosis and would send them to another doctor who would not, or could not, confirm that the patient had lupus. Eventually, the patient would be unemployed because of the illness.

This is a very difficult situation to be in, and there seems to be no best way to handle it. As we assess the matter, it is important to remember that others around us will also deny our illness just as we have done. They may look at the patient and think, "You don't look sick so get on with it!" This is part of life, and though it seems unfair, we must learn to live with it whether we like it or not.

I have talked with a number of lupus patients who are afraid to tell their employers that they have lupus. Pattie and I have talked many times about lupus and how to live with various aspects of the disease. She told me that before she knew that she had lupus she felt that the fluorescent lights she worked under were making her sick. After she was diagnosed with lupus, she wanted to work another three years so that she would be assured of company health insurance. However, her prescription medicine was making her sick, and she quit taking it and denied her illness. She finally was no longer able to continue working and was six months short of her goal. She was then unemployed and without health insurance and other benefits. Her advice to others is, "Don't deny your illness regardless of what it may cost you."

After two attempts to get Social Security, Pattie found it necessary to have an attorney represent her. She was finally granted Social Security because of her disability. As a result of her action with Social Security, and because she had been illegally fired, her company was forced to reinstate her health insurance and give her disability retirement.

As I talked with another lupus patient, she told me that she keeps turning down a promotion and her employer doesn't understand why. I asked her, "Have you told your employer you have lupus and you are afraid that you may not be able to handle the increased pressure of the new position?" She said, "No, I'm afraid that I may lose my job." I asked, "Since he has valued you as an employee worthy of a more responsible position, do you think he would terminate your employment because you have lupus?" She replied, "I don't feel secure in bringing the matter up with him."

One of the problems we face with the employer is that people tend to fear what they don't understand in the matter of diseases. Many have not heard of lupus and fear that it may be another communicable disease. Some employers may have heard that lupus is an immune disease and be afraid it is like AIDS. They need to understand that it is just the opposite. AIDS is a disease in which the immune system isn't working to protect the body. In Lupus the immune system is too active and attacks the body. An allergy is that kind of an over- reaction when the immune system sees an innocent pollen or food as a wicked enemy. Here we can use a bit of humor and say, "I guess my big problem is that I'm allergic to myself, and I must learn to live with it." I have observed that such remarks have a way of easing tensions. It can also be a little bit of fun as someone has said, "Those who can laugh at themselves shall never cease to be amused."

Perhaps that fear could be set aside by stating that lupus is related to arthritis. Many have arthritis to some degree, and it is easy to relate to it. Finding an easy way to educate your employer about the disease and how it affects you and your work may be a good approach. One cannot advise another how they should handle their illness and employment. Every situation is different. However, I do think it is important that the patient talk it over with an understanding friend as a means of self-discovery in how to handle the problem, and then find the courage to act upon what needs to be done.

Some who find it very difficult to work full time and still get the rest they need may be able to work part-time. However, if a person doesn't have to work to support himself/herself, some volunteer work could be beneficial to your health and give the important sense of accomplishment.

I was fortunate to have an employer who I could approach with confidence and know that he would understand. As I worked with my limitations, I discovered that I could spend the morning hours working one area of my territory, go home at noon and rest for an hour, and spend the afternoon working another area. I was fortunate that I could arrange my days the way that suited me best. I was satisfied that I was not neglecting my company or my customers.

The time finally came when the company was making room for another salesman and that meant reshuffling the territories. I must give up some of mine and take some from another. In the reshuffle, my field manager thought he was doing what was best for me. However, it would have been better if he had discussed the matter with me rather than making an executive decision.

As it turned out, I lost two-thirds of my good territory and gained a few good customers from another salesman. I have always enjoyed making new friends and also exploring new territory so that was a plus factor, but trying to find new customers required more energy.

After working the new territory for about three months, I decided that I should make a long-term evaluation of my work and my health. Some of the thoughts I was wrestling with were that the economy had plunged into a deep recession and since my earnings were based on my sales, my income was not as good as it had been. The territory looked good for sales, but I didn't have the strength to develop it. I was no longer able to go home and rest during the noon hour. I was also facing retirement within three years. If I decided to work three more years, my retirement pay would be considerably better. After pondering the issues for a while, I chose early retirement as the best course of action. However, that was not an easy decision.

Before I retired I thought that if I was going to be happy in retirement I should be determined to:

1. Live within my income regardless of the changes life demanded.
2. Find a way to be of service to my community.
3. Encourage others in need and help them in their struggles.

I needed to be involved in something that would be meaningful to me and also benefit others.

As I look back on my twelve years of retirement, I realize that I could not have developed a better philosophy for the years ahead. It wasn't easy adjusting to not going to work each day. We had moved to our mountain home, and it was winter and I couldn't do the things outside that I wanted to get done. Consequently, I was developing a full blown case of "cabin fever" until someone called and wanted some photographs made. I was busy with promotional photographs for that company for the remainder of the year, which helped to bridge the gap between employment and retirement. Now I often wonder; "When did I ever have time to work?"

I realize that every work situation has its advantages and disadvantages and the patient is faced with the desire to be productive and earn a livelihood. At times work may seem like drudgery; however, it is God's gift to us.[2] We need to work, not just for the income, but to fulfill the need of meaning and purpose in life. All of us have skills and abilities and the need to express and use them.

Jerry, a friend of mine, was deliberately run down by an angry driver. His life hung in the balance for several weeks. After a year of therapy and recuperation, he returned to work. Within a few months, he felt that his superiors were trying to force him into disability retirement. His retirement income would have been better than the wages many others earn—but he didn't want to retire!

---

2 Ecclesiastes 2:24

One could rationalize and conclude that he should seize the opportunity. He would have a decent income and would be free to pursue other interests. His wife, Jodi, owns a race car, and Jerry drives it. Think of all the racing he could do.

Jerry likes to keep his priorities in order. For him, auto racing is a sport, and he won't let it consume him. As we were discussing the alternatives, Jerry said, "I have abilities and skills that I want to continue using. I like my work and don't want to retire." He is continuing to resist being forced into disability retirement.

I have used these illustrations to show the traumatic feelings the patient faces at the threat of the loss of employment. The loss of income, or a drastically reduced income, is a major consideration and may keep us from exploring other avenues of life. Our identity is often attached to our work, and a basic need is to feel needed and to know that we are fulfilling our role in life. However, if the patient can live on a drastically reduced income, there are ways to fulfill our deeper needs and enjoy a productive and joyful adventure. There is hope, and I encourage you to explore all of the possibilities. You may be surprised at what life has to offer!

Chapter 14

The Adventure of Faith

"Now faith is being sure of what we hope for and certain of what we do not see."[1]

Once again, as we think of adventure, we must remember that an adventure is not static or routine. Adventure requires a commitment to explore new territory. One does not know exactly the turns it may take, the dangers involved, the hardships that may be encountered, or even what the outcome may be. However, the person must be committed to it and persevere to its completion.

When we think of faith and illness, many think of being healed through their faith. Sometimes a person is told, "If you only had enough faith, you would be healed of your illness." The person who

---

[1] Hebrews 11:1, New International Version

makes such a remark reveals that either he does not understand faith or he doesn't know what to say. I do believe there are some who are miraculously healed in answer to prayer, while there are many others who are not. Does that mean that those who are not healed do not have faith?

There have been a few times during my life that I have seen people miraculously healed in answer to prayer. I recall a time when a woman asked a group of us to meet at the church to pray for her niece who had been stricken with spinal meningitis. Her niece lived in a town a few hundred miles from us. That was a prayer meeting I shall never forget. We prayed for a long while, one after another. Each one prayed several times, and suddenly there was no longer a burden to pray. We all felt that our prayers were answered. The next day the girl's mother called and said she had just returned from the hospital. The doctor was mystified; he could not find a trace of spinal meningitis in the girl's body. God answered our prayers, and the girl was healed.

A lady called one evening and requested the elders of the church to anoint her with oil and pray for her healing. We gathered around her bed and read to her from the Book of James, "Are any among you sick? They should call for the elders of the church and have them pray over them, anointing them with oil in the name of the Lord. The prayer of faith will save the sick, and the Lord will raise them up; and anyone who has committed sins will be forgiven. Therefore confess your sins to one another, and pray for one another, so that you may be healed. The prayer of the righteous is powerful and effective."[2]

---

[2] James 5:13-18, New Standard Revised Version

After we read the Scripture to the lady we asked if she had searched her heart concerning her relationship to God and others, and if there was anything she was aware of that should be made right. She assured us that she had done that and knew of no reason why God should not heal her. We anointed her with oil and prayed for her. At her next doctor's appointment the doctor said, "I don't understand this. I don't find anything wrong with you." The lady later told us that while we were praying for her she could feel changes taking place in her body.

I could cite other times when people have been healed in direct answer to prayer. I could also show many other occasions when nothing physical happened; however, the spiritual lives of the individuals involved were deepened.

The Apostle Paul, who God used so greatly, said, "To keep me from becoming conceited because of these surpassingly great revelations, there was given me a thorn in my flesh...three times I pleaded with the Lord to take it away from me. But he said to me, `My grace is sufficient for you.'"[3] Paul also wrote about faith and spiritual gifts, and one of the gifts of the Spirit is that of healing, yet he was not healed of his own affliction. Though God had healed others through Paul's ministry, God's grace was sufficient for him to live with his own affliction.

It is important that we understand that not everyone who prays is going to be physically healed. When I first came down with lupus, I searched the

---

[3] 2 Corinthians 12:7-9, New International Version

Scriptures and my heart in this regard. I also went
to the library, eventually checked out every book I
could find on faith healing, and read them all.
Some of them were shallow; some were deep.
Some made sense, while others left me wondering.
I think I explored the full gamut of faith healing.
Even though I prayed for healing, nothing seemed
to change. Others prayed for me, and it didn't
appear to make any difference. Was it that I didn't
have faith? No.   Faith trusts God even though
He does not seem to answer our prayers. In the
Book of Psalms, the psalmist expresses time and
again that God does not seem to hear his prayers. At
other times there is great rejoicing because of what
God has done in answer to prayer. Job expresses
anguish because he could not understand his
suffering and why God was silent. In his
bewilderment he said, "Though he slay me, yet I
will hope in him."[4]

It is interesting to note that here in the Book of
Job, God reveals Job's lowest and highest points
right next to each other. This same God has created
the highest and lowest elevations in California that
can be seen from the same spot.

My wife and I were looking across Death Valley
where the elevation is 282 feet below sea level. We
looked beyond that point and saw Mount Whitney
with an elevation of 14,494 feet above sea level.

Job, from the depth of his suffering, has given us
great statements of faith that have comforted and
strengthened others ever since. When we are at our
lowest point in life, we must remember that God

---

[4] Job 13:15, New International Version

has not forsaken us. We can look across our valley of despair and see the mount of God's blessing standing high before us.

The person who has faith in God must not believe that there will never be adverse experiences in life. When we read the eleventh chapter of Hebrews we discover the hardships that many believers endured. You can also read the history of the early church and discover that Christians went through unmerciful persecution and suffered, even horrible deaths, for no other reason than that they were followers of Christ. During World War II Hitler unleashed his hatred upon the Jews and also the Christians. While the Iron Curtain was in place in the Soviet Union, the believers in Christ suffered untold hardships. Raisa Gorbachev in her book, *I Hope*, says that the Iron Curtain subdued the expression of faith. That is true; however, it is also stating it lightly.

We must remember that as long as we are in this world there will be sickness, pain, and suffering. Just because a person claims to have faith in Christ does not make him or her immune to ill health or pain and suffering. Some of the greatest lessons of life are learned during the most serious times of illness or hard trials.

Bernie Siegle in his book, *Peace, Love & Healing*, raises the question, "Why do you need your illness?" If it had not been for my last three months of being in bed during a lupus flare, I would not have an appreciation of the "wisdom of God" that I have today. I have a clearer understanding of anger and its effect upon me as well as upon others around me and also how to control it in a more gracious manner. It is through the hardships of life that these most important things are brought into focus. Yes, it may sound strange, but I needed my illness!

The Apostle Paul also needed his "thorn in [the] flesh." He said it was "To keep me from becoming conceited because of these surpassingly great revelations [God had given him] there was given me a thorn in my flesh...to torment me."[5] His greatest need was a spiritual one that he learned through suffering. You might also ask, "Why do I need my illness?" If you can properly answer that question, life may dramatically change for you. That does not mean we like it or want it, but it does mean that we can live with it and benefit from it.

The Prophet Isaiah wrote, "'For my thoughts are not your thoughts, neither are your ways my ways;' declares the Lord. 'As the heavens are higher than the earth, so are my ways higher than your ways and my thoughts than your thoughts.'"[6] In the depths of our illness, we must not think that when we pray for healing and are not healed that God is indifferent to us. I was in a prayer group as we prayed for a child with a terminal illness. As one man prayed, he commanded God to heal the boy. This is not a true expression of "bold faith"; neither is it an example of how to pray.

When we pray, we should not attempt to bend God's ways and thoughts to ours. He is the Sovereign God and we are to align our lives with His. It is better to ask, "Sovereign God, what do you

---

[5] 2 Corinthians 12:7, New International Version

[6] Isaiah 55:8-9, New International Version

want me to learn in this trial that I am going through?" You may need to seek the counsel of a Christian friend to help you though your trial. Choose a friend who can feel your anxieties and sit with you, rather than impose his or her values upon you and cause further anxiety.

I am fortunate that I have had a long-time experience in the Christian faith; however, I still needed the help, support, and encouragement of other Christians. I shall never forget one experience when I started making sales calls after about four months absence. I was in the electrical harness department at Douglas Aircraft, and while seated and waiting, I was softly singing, "I don't know about tomorrow...but I know Who holds my hand...." A lady came up to me and said, "I heard your song, and I want you to know that because of your long absence I thought you must have been seriously ill, and I have been praying for you." What a lift that gave me! Talk about encouragement! Even in the marketplace, nothing could have been more apropos for the moment. I was literally living just one day at a time. I could not think of tomorrow or try to borrow from it.

Faith is taking God at His word and demonstrating it by obedience to Him. The eleventh chapter of Hebrews has often been referred to as the "hall of fame" because it tells how faith has changed the lives of so many individuals, regardless of the difficulties they were called upon to endure. The very heart of that faith is stated in verse six, "And without faith it is impossible to please God, because anyone who comes to him must believe that he exists and that he rewards those who earnestly seek him." We must also remember that those spoken of experienced hardships and adverse times just as we do. However, God blessed them in many ways and "All these people were still living by faith when they died. They did not receive the things promised; they only saw them and welcomed them from a distance." The Scriptures go on to say; "They admitted that they were aliens and strangers on earth. People who say such things show that they are looking for a country of their own...they were longing for a better country—a heavenly one. Therefore God is not ashamed to be called their God, for he has prepared a city for them."[7]

At no time can I say that I have enjoyed my illness. I have said that I needed it so that I could see life from another perspective. I have also realized that my greatest need for healing has been not in the physical aspects of life, but the spiritual.

Looking back over my seventy-five years of life, my journey of faith has had its ups and downs, times of great joy and times of disappointment. However, the greatest lessons have been learned under the most difficult circumstances of life. The lessons learned are what makes the adventure a wonderful experience.

Ever since the last time I spent three months in bed with a lupus flare, I can say that the ensuing years have been some of the richest of my life. I am able to relate to the younger generation, even the junior high age, and also to adults of all ages to encourage them in their personal lives. Though my

---

[7] Hebrews 11:13-16, New International Version

lupus has been in remission for more than three years, I am active in a support group to support and encourage others who are going down the pathway I have traveled.

Just recently I have added another chapter to my adventure. My wife and I, along with another lupus patient, put on our first Lupus Education Seminar in Bakersfield, California. There was a charge for the seminar. After the materials were paid for, the remainder of the money went to our local support group to help others. It is our desire to give hope to those who find the disease so difficult to understand and often very trying to live with.

When the focus is on *life* rather than on illness, there is hope. In Richard Nixon's book, *In the Arena*, he painfully tells of his resignation from the presidency, his severe physical complications with phlebitis that nearly cost him his life, and the deep depression that he went through. He was given hope through the support of his family and the prayers of many that he will never meet; that is what brought him through. He said that he needed time to heal, physically, spiritually, and mentally. He also stated that the last ten years have been his most creative years. In his final book, *Beyond Peace*, Mr. Nixon says that our country may be rich in goods, but poor in spirit. Raisa Gorbachev made a similar observation in her book, *I Hope*.

It is interesting to note that people at the seat of power from two great nations that have different ideologies would make similar observations; that the material aspects of life can not satisfy the deepest needs of mankind, which are spiritual. Both have made this observation through struggling with the hardships of life.

I believe that as we experience the adversities of life, and put them in proper perspective, our lives will be richer than before. So, when this becomes our experience and we think there is no hope, remember that we are not alone, and along with others who have been where we are, we can say also, "I *choose* to live!"

My personal journey has taken me over steep and rugged pathways that have sapped my strength and at times discouragement almost got the best of me as the "wolf" dogged my trail. During that long and lonely journey, I learned to respect the "wolf" in his natural environment, and he began to keep his distance. By the grace of God, I have entered the clearing at the edge of the wilderness and am now free of the "wolf."

Chapter 14

A Nurse's Viewpoint

By Beth Yocum R.N.

THE PAST

As a child I was surrounded by chronic illnesses though of course I wasn't aware of it at the time. It seemed to be a normal part of life. When I was five, my mother was sickly and was finally diagnosed with tuberculosis. She was in hospitals, sanitariums and private care until I was about thirteen. Mom was still weak and my older brother and I helped with the housework. That was a normal part of life too. Mom had one lung that had been permanently collapsed and it was hard for her to get enough oxygen. In later years she developed heart trouble, emphysema, San Joaquin Valley Fever, and severe anemia but lived to celebrate her sixtieth wedding anniversary.

In the meantime, I had been living back and forth between my grandparents (all of my relatives lived in Ventura County, Southern California). None of them was really healthy. My paternal grandmother had been crippled since she was thirteen, but raised a family of six children, and then grandchildren. My paternal grandfather had diabetes which resulted in his death when I was ten years old. He was the only one of my grandparents (or parents) who didn't live into his eighties.

My maternal grandmother had a bad heart. I remember hearing when I was a child that she had been told twenty years before that she wouldn't live long unless she learned to take it easy. Well, she never learned to take it easy and lived until shortly before our first child was born. I vividly remember one time when she had an attack and sent me out to the edge of the hill to ring a cowbell to call my grandfather who was working in the orchard below. He was reasonably healthy and a hard worker until later years.

My father's sister helped raise me though she was just four years older than I was. When we were at my grandmother's cottage at Hueneme, Mary taught me to swim in the ocean where there was sometimes a riptide. Her chronic illness was epilepsy, but I don't remember when it first bothered her. She still takes medication for it.

After high school and two years at Ventura Junior College, I went to work in the office at the Port Hueneme Naval Base and lived in my grandmother's little cottage. However, I had always wanted to be a nurse and with the war on, that seemed to be a very necessary occupation. Once on the Greyhound bus going home for the weekend, I sat with Maria whom I had known in junior college. She was in nurses' training at a hospital in Los Angeles and told me she thought I might be able to get into the nurses' program at the Los Angeles County General Hospital, even though I hadn't taken the proper preliminary courses in junior college.

It rather surprised me when I applied and was accepted, and if I hadn't taken that step, I would never have met Bob. I think the Lord put Maria and me together as part of his plan for me. For the next three years I lived in the nurses' cottages and worked and learned at the L.A. County Hospital. The Lord also sent Gevene Robinson, who was in an upper class, and Edna Thiesen, my next door neighbor, to be my best friends. Edna had graduated from BIOLA (the Bible Institute of Los Angeles) and was preparing to be a missionary. Gevene was also preparing for missionary service and worked at it right where she was, starting a nurses' weekly chapel service and later a nurses' Bible study under the Navigators. Like Bob, she was a very energetic person.

One memorable day we had gone to a meeting at Gevene's family home in Pasadena. Gevene's brother, Bob, a tall nice-looking sailor, was home on leave, and after the meeting, Bob offered to drive us back to the hospital. We had a curfew but had plenty of time so stopped on the way to get something to eat. Bob was a charming, fun person to be around. That impressed me because I was rather shy and basically serious minded. I did like him very much but knew nothing would come of it as our lives were headed in different directions. One drawback was that he smoked, but the main problem was that he wasn't a Christian and wasn't headed for the mission field.

Bob went back to sea, and Gevene would intermittently tell us about him. Then came the day we heard his destroyer had been hit by a suicide plane and had limped back to Long Beach for repairs. I learned that since I'd met him he had given his life to the Lord. After his discharge from the Navy he started taking the three-year Missionary Course at BIOLA, but we had no real contact. We sometimes attended Youth for Christ and various youth activities and saw each other in passing. I heard that he was dating another nursing student, but I guess that didn't last long.

After a time we sort of paired off, though still in a group, and later began dating seriously. It seemed that now our lives were heading in the same direction and since we both felt that the Lord had brought us together, we were married in June, 1947.

Our daughter, Audrey, was born the following June. We seriously considered going to South America as missionaries but never had any clear leading from the Lord. Then we had an opportunity to work in a Christian camp in Wyoming for the summer so off we went. That led to the pastorate of a small church in Manderson, Wyoming for a year. Bob decided he needed to go back to school and get his college degree, so when our second child, Sam, was three months old, we returned to Southern California and Bob returned to BIOLA.

Trying to learn Greek and study the other subjects at BIOLA, as well as working on the side, was giving Bob ulcers, so it seemed expedient to accept the call to a small pastorate in the little town of Ramona in San Diego County. A major accomplishment was building their first church building. Our third and last child, Russell, was born there; in fact, we celebrated his first birthday a week after moving to Oxnard where we built another church.

Our story almost ended right there as we almost didn't make it to Oxnard. We were moving, driving up the coast road with high cliffs towering on our right. Some young fellows who had been drinking were speeding and tried to pass us on a curve. They were going too fast to get around us on the left so tried to pass on the right and their car went right up the cliff and out of sight above us. Debris from the cliff was falling on our car, and I said to myself "Lord, here we come!" but we didn't.

I would have continued driving or put on the brake and waited for that car to come down on top of us, but Bob was a much more experienced driver. He stepped on the gas and headed for the opposite side of the road. Fortunately, no cars were coming and we were in the clear. The car crashed on the road behind us scattering bodies on the road. One of the young men was killed, but the other two recovered after extended hospitalization. The five of us were uninjured, and our car wasn't even scratched. We decided the Lord wasn't through with us and had work for us to do.

Our final church was in Long Beach where the area was changing rapidly. Whites were moving out and black people, Latinos and South East Asians were moving in. We encouraged a black group to hold church services in our building at alternate hours, and as our congregation moved away, we turned the building over to the new group. That left Bob without a church to work in, and since he was already working on the side, he continued as a salesman for Snap-On Tools.

When Bob got sick, we had already bought property in the Tehachapi Mountains and had begun building our retirement home there. After being diagnosed and treated for lupus and finding he just didn't have the strength and energy he'd always had, he decided to take early retirement and we moved to our new home in the Tehachapi Valley. Gevene, who first brought us together, was retiring as a missionary in Mexico so we built an apartment for her connected to our house.

Retiring was rather traumatic for Bob who had been working for a living since he was sixteen. He didn't know what he was going to do with himself and couldn't see himself sitting in a rocking chair taking it easy. There were things to finish on the house, and he kept adding on. The two car garage never housed a car and was soon turned into an office. He built a carport, a couple of tool sheds, a wood shed, and enclosed the back porch. He put turbo-chargers in a pickup truck, and he would take the dog up to the mountains and cut wood for the wood stove. We have an acre of ground, and there is a lot of work to do in the yard.

Bob had built a darkroom into the house and expanded his photographic equipment and capabilities.

He took up oil painting, and I can look up and see some of his pictures on the walls. He has been busy at church and in various civic projects. He started learning about computers and is on his fourth computer now.

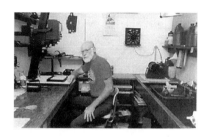

Photography is a gratifying hobby that I have enjoyed over the years, and it is my only duty at the races. This is my dark room.

Another thing he really enjoyed was rebuilding his old BSA motorcycle that was nothing but frame. He bought what parts he could, some Harley and some Kawasaki parts and whatever else would fit, and made some parts from whatever was at hand. He painted it beautifully and painted a helmet to match, and it attracts attention wherever he goes.

Like Bob, most people who have lupus are very energetic, type A personalities. Idleness isn't in their makeup. If they have a job that isn't too strenuous, they may be better off working and keeping busy. If a job isn't feasible, they need to find some other interests to keep their minds occupied. It's bad for a person to sit and feel sorry for themselves.

Bob is still fun to be with and has a good sense of humor. We have talked about the fact that "laughter is the best medicine," or as the Living Bible version of Proverbs 17:22 says, "A cheerful heart does good like medicine, but a broken spirit makes one sick." You may get annoyed with people telling you to cheer up or to keep a positive outlook, but if it's good medicine, why not do it. Norman Cousins told of using laughter as a medicine. He would get comedy films to watch and found that laughing really made him better. You might find it helpful too.

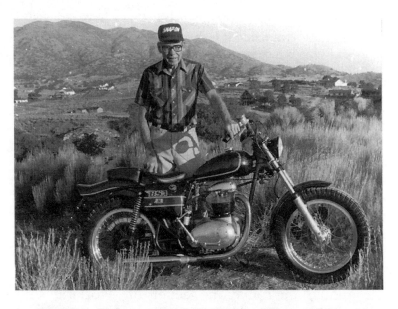

My BSA. This motorcycle just grew. Whenever I could find parts I used them to construct this bike. It is a combination of Kawasaki, Suzuki, Harley Davidson, BSA and specially-fabricated components

One of Bob's desirable traits is that he enjoys helping people. Sometimes he helps young people with photography and learning to develop and print pictures in his darkroom. He has helped others who are just trying to learn to use a computer. He has assisted some in writing special letters or nice-looking resumes to apply for a job. When the shoe is on the other foot and he has to accept help from someone else, he is uncomfortable. He didn't know how to react when a neighbor mowed our lawn, or a friend cut up wood for our stove.

Just this morning Bob was at his computer making some revisions on this book when a friend came by. He had a problem and needed someone to talk to. As usual, Bob dropped what he was doing and helped someone else. It is not unusual for people to come to Bob for advice. I think that helping and encouraging people are good therapies too.

THE FUTURE

As a nurse, I have been very interested in learning all I can about lupus—its causes, treatment, and potential future treatments. Much work and research are being done into both auto-immune diseases and genetics. One of the best books I have read on lupus is *Living with Lupus* by Sheldon Paul Blau, M.D. and Dodi Schultz. It tells what lupus is, possible causes, medications and other treatments, hope for the future, etc., and it is very readable. It answers many of the questions you might have.

We found that libraries didn't seem to have much information on lupus. Besides books, the best place to get current information is from the Lupus Foundation of America. We joined the Bay Area Lupus Foundation, so we receive their three newsletters each year as well as three newsletters from the National Lupus Foundation. They have very informative articles. The Lupus Group also has informative classes and can answer questions people have.

When we first learned that Bob had lupus, it was called a connective tissue disease. Later it was termed a collagen disease, and now is usually referred to as an auto-immune disease, one in which white cells in your body attack your own body and/or specific parts of it.

I was amazed to learn that many other diseases such as rheumatoid arthritis, auto-immune thyroid, multiple sclerosis, myasthenia gravis, scleroderma, Behcet's syndrome, Sjogren's syndrome, insulin-dependent diabetes, chronic fatigue syndrome, ankylosing spondylitis (Norman Cousin's disease) and allergies are all now considered to be auto-immune diseases. It was also amazing that lupus is more prevalent than multiple sclerosis which gets much more publicity.

As parents, one of our first concerns was "Will my children inherit this disease?" It is true that 10 percent of lupus patients have close relatives with lupus. Bob's mother had lupus, and though generally lupus is more prevalent in young women in their child-bearing years, she wasn't diagnosed until she was over sixty. It wasn't recognized, diagnosed, and treated early so her heart was affected and her heart finally killed her at the age of eighty-three. Other relatives might develop another auto-immune disease such as rheumatoid arthritis.

I tell you this, not to frighten you, but so you will be aware and seek early diagnosis of any symptoms in your children that might be suspicious. Many people have been sick for years before the diagnosis of lupus was finally made, but the tests are getting better and most doctors are learning more about lupus and other auto-immune diseases. One lady we know who has lupus has a young daughter who has been diagnosed as having juvenile arthritis. Both are getting along very well and are able to live nearly normal lives.

More research is being done into auto-immune diseases and new treatments are being tried. Genetic therapy is also making great strides. No gene has been isolated for lupus, and it is possible that you may have to have a combination of several genes before you can get the disease. And just because you have those genes, doesn't mean that you have to get the disease. It usually takes some other trigger to bring it on. I think it was stress associated with a serious surgery that brought on Bob's lupus.

The good news is that there are new treatments in your future. Testing is getting better for early diagnosis. You have every reason to hope and expect that things will get better. Work with your doctor, and if one medication isn't working or doesn't agree with you, ask for an alternate. Write down your symptoms and any problems with medications before you visit your doctor. If you are like me, your mind tends to go blank when the doctor comes in and asks, "How are you feeling?"

Do you have a tendency to say "fine" whether it's true or not? My mind also goes blank when I walk into a grocery store without a list.

Some of the medications such as prednisone can seem to be miracle drugs and make you feel like a new person immediately. But the anti-malarials such as Plaquenil take several months to take effect so don't be discouraged. It was interesting to me to learn that during World War II Atabrine was given to servicemen in the South Pacific to prevent malaria (Bob would never take his; it turned everyone yellow, and he claimed mosquitoes never bit him anyway). It was discovered that the men's joint pains got better when taking the anti-malarial medication.

These medications can cause serious side effects so should be taken only under careful monitoring by your doctor. If you have a problem with the prescribed medication, don't just stop taking it; some need to be tapered off. Phone your doctor and talk it over immediately. If you can't get through to him, ask to talk to his nurse (not the receptionist). The nurse can be a good intermediary.

If all else fails, find a new doctor who will listen to you. Be sure you have one primary care doctor who is aware of any treatments or medications that specialists may be giving you. Some lupus patients go to several different doctors for different problems, and it's important to have one doctor who is sent reports from all of them and can coordinate treatment. Many lupus patients choose to go to a rheumatologist who specializes in diseases such as rheumatoid arthritis and lupus. We chose to stay with a knowledgeable internist in our own community rather than drive an hour each way to a specialist. She refers us to specialists if it seems necessary. Recently she sent Bob to a cardiologist because of a heart murmur she noticed at his last physical. Results of the tests are sent to her.

Bob doesn't think that sunlight and fluorescent lighting bother him, but there was at least one time when it did. He was with his sister in a large home supply store which had fluorescent lighting, and when it came time to leave, he couldn't find his way out. The fluorescent lighting seemed to make him disoriented, and if Gevene hadn't been with him, he wouldn't have been able to find the exit or the car. Such disorientation is not really uncommon, so don't be too upset if it happens to you. But be aware that fluorescent lighting might be the cause.

We can't stress enough the importance of a support group and a support person who will listen to you and understand. It may be your spouse, but if not, find someone you can talk to or call on the phone who will understand. It may be helpful to have another lupus patient to talk to because that person can understand your problems and can encourage you. Urge your spouse and teen-age children to attend the support group once in a while. They need to understand lupus too.

If you get to the place where you can be an encouragement and help to someone else, it will also do you a world of good. Learn to avoid unnecessary stress, and try to look at the bright side. I've read that people with lupus seldom have cancer. Though you may have painful joints, you aren't apt to have deformed joints as is true of many people with arthritis.

So which would you rather have, lupus or cancer? I would rather have lupus than be crippled as my grandmother was or be blind as Bob's grandmother was. Think of all the horrible diseases you could have, and learn to be thankful that you only have lupus.

Epilogue

The adventure continues. Working with publishers has become another part of the adventure. I have been rejected by some and verbally dismissed by another. However, when I received a phone call from Griffin Publishing, the adventure took on new meaning, especially when asked if I would add more to the manuscript.

After about four years of freedom from the wolf, there are times when I have wondered if I am hearing its howl once again. As I cautiously wait, I can only conclude that it is an echo from the past.

Writing this book has been not only an adventure, but also it has been therapeutic. I believe this whole experience has been a major factor for being in remission today. Ruth Vaughn in her book, *Write to Discover Yourself*, speaks of how creative writing helps us to focus our thoughts and feelings. I believe that has been one of my greatest benefits from writing the book. It has helped me to remove the blurry thoughts and feelings about my illness and take positive steps and attitudes toward wellness.

Through my many start and stop experiences, I often thought, "If I never finish the book, or it is never published, what I have written has been of great benefit to me because I understand myself better than I had before.

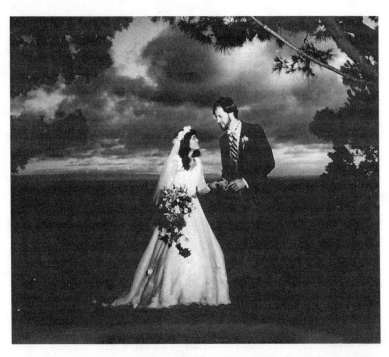

Russell and Suzie's wedding. The spectacular photograph was taken in a natural setting

As I have stated previously, I was often compelled to take up my pen once again when someone was helped and encouraged by what I had written. Even now, I thought the book had been completed until the publisher asked me to add more to it. I like that!

It gives me the feeling that my adventure has become a part of their adventure.

In 1981 I was discouraged, depressed and ready to give up. Living with lupus has been an experience totally different from any other experience during my life. I am glad I didn't give up as I now see all that I would have missed.

I have had the privilege of encouraging many other lupus patients. I have helped in the establishment of a helpful support group and the development of an annual educational seminar. It is also gratifying to see others becoming more involved in the work to help others learn to live with their illness.

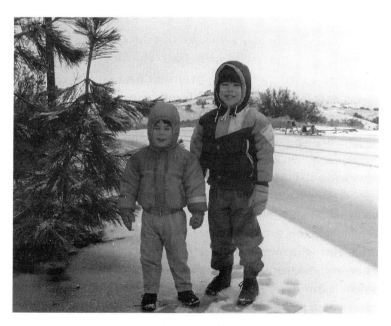

Stephen and Ryan

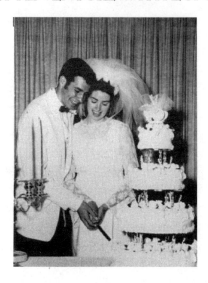

Michael & Audrey's wedding

If I had given up, I would not have seen my son Russell get married nor had the joy of being a grandpa to his two sons, Stephen and Ryan. I would have missed Stephen's enjoyable adventure of his first few days away from home without his parents, at grandpa's house.

Stephen would have been deprived of some precious memories such as a good water fight with his grandpa, the closeness at bedtime when grandpa would read him a story and then pretend to be reading from a book while making up a story. What was the impression it made on him? The next evening Stephen climbed into bed with me and said, "Grandpa, read me a story out of the book, and then read me a story out of your hands." Isn't that a heartwarming experience!

One should never give up! If I had, I would have missed my grandson Joshua's wedding. His oldest daughter, Christa would have missed a special time with her great-grandpa. While she was taking a nap after a good lunch and an afternoon in the park, Beth and I left for home. When Christa awakened she said to her grandma, Audrey, "I have two grandpas and two grandmas, a great-grandma and a great-grandpa, and he's my friend!"

Both Stephen and Ryan love their grandparents, and Christa and Ariel love their great grandparents. Being a grandparent is a wonderful experience and it also affords the opportunity to give good memories to our grandchildren and also to help instill good values that we hope they will treasure during their growing experience.

Never give up! Never stop learning! In 1957 I was given a book, *How to Live 365 Days A Year*. The book is about emotionally induced illnesses and ways to avoid them. In Chapter 13, the author addresses "senility." In his view, senility is mainly the result of mental laziness. He believes that the mind is intended to grow as long as the person is alive. Since then I have also read other doctors and psychologists who have made similar observations. That has been a vital part of my adventure.

If I had given up and neglected that aspect of life, I would not have owned four different computers. Some have remarked that my accomplishment with the computer is remarkable for a man my age. I must confess that I have found it intimidating, frustrating and also challenging. The computer has challenged me to continue learning something new. There seems to be no end to that challenge since there is something entirely new that is developed every twenty minutes, so they say.

No, I haven't given up and have no intention of doing so. I can honestly say that I enjoy the frustrating experience of learning a new computer program. My computer is not just for my entertainment and learning; it is also an instrument I use to help and benefit others.

Yes, as the adventure continues, I find it as exciting now as at other times. It is my hope and desire that through sharing my adventure with you that you will find encouragement in your trials of life. If I had given up, as I was tempted to do, or felt sorry for myself and murmured and complained, I would have never experienced some of the greatest years of my life. May the God of all comfort, Who has comforted me in my time of trouble, comfort you as you face your trials of life.